your pregnancy™

Quick Guide

Feeding Your Baby in the First Year

your
pregnancy™
Quick Guide

Feeding Your Baby in the First Year

Glade B. Curtis, M.D., M.P.H., OB-GYN

Judith Schuler, M.S.

Da Capo

LIFE
LONG

A Member of the Perseus Books Group

Designed by Brent Wilcox
Set in 11.5-point Minion by The Perseus Books Group

First printing, 2004

Library of Congress Cataloging-in-Publication data

Curtis, Glade B.
    Your pregnancy quick guide : feeding your baby in the first year / Glade B. Curtis and Judith Schuler.
        p. cm.
    Includes index.
    ISBN 0-7382-0968-6 (pbk. : alk. paper)
    1. Infants—Nutrition. 2. Breast feeding.   3. Bottle feeding.   4. Baby foods. I. Schuler, Judith.   II. Title.
RJ216.C875 2004
649'.33—dc22

                                                                        2004016199

Published by Da Capo Press
A Member of the Perseus Books Group
http://www.dacapopress.com

Note: The information in this book is true and complete to the best of our knowledge. The book is intended only as an informative guide for those wishing to know more about feeding a baby during the first year. In no way is this book intended to replace, countermand, or conflict with the advice given to you by your baby's pediatrician. The ultimate decision concerning your care and your baby's care should be made between you and your doctors. We strongly recommend that you follow their advice. The information in this book is general and is offered with no guarantees on the part of the authors or Da Capo Press. The authors and publisher disclaim all liability in connection with the use of this book. The names and identifying details of people associated with events described in this book have been changed. Any similarity to actual persons is coincidental.

Da Capo Press books are available at special discounts for bulk purchases in the U.S. by corporations, institutions, and other organizations. For more information, please contact the Special Markets Department at the Perseus Books Group, 11 Cambridge Center, Cambridge, MA 02142, or call (800) 255-1514 or (617) 252-5298, or email special.markets@perseusbooks.com.

2 3 4 5 6 7 8 9—08 07 06 05 04

Find It Fast!

Part IV: Beyond the Breast and Bottle—
It's Time to Feed Baby Solids

Giving Your Baby the Best Start

Feeding your baby is one of the most important tasks you will perform. The nutrition you give your baby *now* will have an effect on the rest of his or her life. You want to help give your baby the best start nutritionally that you can. If you any have questions, discuss them with your baby's pediatrician or your doctor. It helps if you work together as a team in this important undertaking.

In this book, we discuss bottlefeeding, breastfeeding, feeding your baby solids, and situations and problems that may come while feeding your baby this first year. The information we provide will help you make decisions during baby's first year.

You may decide to breastfeed baby; it's probably the best nutrition you can give your new baby. The baby receives more than just breast milk from you. He or she will also receive important nutrients, antibodies to help prevent infections and other substances that are important for growth and development. However, you may choose not to breastfeed—if you bottlefeed, you can still provide good nutrition for your baby.

Note: In each section, we will use one gender for baby. In the following section, we will use the opposite gender. We hope this will make reading the material a little easier.

Part I: General Guidelines for Feeding Your Baby

You may feel uncertain when you think about feeding your baby. How will you know he's hungry? How will you know when he's full? How will you know he's getting enough to eat? How often should you feed him? These important questions (and probably others you haven't even thought about!) will be answered in this book.

Even though this task may be one you're unsure about, your baby will help you. He'll tell you many things, in his own way. You'll know when he's hungry; he'll exhibit definite signs of hunger, including fussing, putting his hands in his mouth and turning his head and opening his mouth when his cheek is touched. You may decide you want to feed at regular intervals to help your baby get on a schedule. Or you may decide to let your baby set his own schedule—some babies need to eat more often than others. Below are some general guidelines.

- Most newborns eat every 3 to 4 hours, although some feed as often as every 2 hours.
- Sometimes, a baby needs to feed more often than usual, such as during periods of growth.
- A baby is usually the best judge of how much he needs at each feeding. He'll usually turn away from the nipple (mother or bottle) when he's full.

- It's a good idea to burp your baby after each feeding. Some babies even need to be burped during a feeding.
- Hold your baby over your shoulder or sit your baby in your lap, and gently rub or pat his back. You will probably want to place a towel over your shoulder or at least have one handy in case he spits up. If your baby doesn't burp, don't force it.
- Babies frequently spit up some breast milk or formula after a feeding. It's common in the early months because the muscle at the top of the stomach is not fully developed.
- When a baby spits up enough to propel the stomach contents several inches, it is called *vomiting*. If your baby vomits after a feeding, don't feed him again immediately. His tummy may be upset; wait until the next feeding.
- If you have questions about baby's feeding, talk to your pediatrician.

Your Partner's Involvement in Feeding Baby

The decision of how baby is fed is one that most new fathers leave to the mother. After all, you're the one who will be involved with feeding the baby, so what kind of input can a father actually have, right? Well, according to researchers, your partner's input matters a lot.

- Studies show that the most common reason a woman gives up breastfeeding her baby is her partner's attitude.

FROM A MOM'S PERSPECTIVE

When I had twins, one was ill and couldn't feed as well as her sister, who was a regular little pig! My doctor suggested I pump my breasts and feed them the breast milk in bottles. That way I could divide up my milk so that each baby got the same amount. To finish off each feeding, I fed them formula after they finished the breast milk. They did real well. I kept pumping my breasts and feeding them this way for about 4 months. *Kim*

- One report indicated that over 75% of all men decide *before* pregnancy or during the *first trimester* whether they want their partner to breastfeed.
- One reason for stopping breastfeeding cited by the men is that they were afraid how society would view their partner if she breastfed in public.

The good news is that when many of these men were made aware of the nutritional and health benefits to baby that breastfeeding provides, they changed their attitudes and supported their partners. Discuss breastfeeding with your partner during your pregnancy. Ask him to support you in whatever you decide to do; he can support you and help with whatever choice you make.

- If you are breastfeeding, your partner can help out at night by getting up and bringing baby to you to nurse. He may even give baby a bottle of expressed breast milk.
- If you bottlefeed, he can take over some of the feedings—you can even switch off for night feedings.

• Involve your partner in this important decision, and ask for his help and support.

Feeding Facts

Just after birth, your baby will probably eat very often. It may help your baby if you get him on a regular schedule. You can do this by timing his feedings. Or you may decide to let baby set his own schedule; some babies need to feed more often. See how often your baby wants to feed and whether he is growing properly. These are the best feeding guides.

• As baby grows older, he usually waits longer between feedings and feeds longer at each feeding.

• A baby is usually the best judge of how much he should take at each feeding. Usually a baby will let you know when he's full, such as by turning away from the nipple.

• Some mothers want to know if it is OK to give baby water sometimes. Discuss it with your baby's doctor. Much depends on your baby's weight, how well he is doing and whether he is hungry or thirsty.

• Most young babies do not need extra fluid. Breast milk and formula contain enough water.

• Too much water can dilute a baby's blood, which could cause sodium and/or electrolyte levels to fall, sometimes dangerously. In severe cases, giving too much water has caused seizures and coma in infants.

My baby was a lazy little guy! He just couldn't be bothered to suck very much. When we went to his 2-week checkup, he hadn't even gained back to his birth weight. I was worried and asked what I should do. My doctor explained to me that a few babies just won't breastfeed hard enough if they get a bottle early. I had been sick, and we had to bottlefeed him formula when I was taking medicine. I tried breastfeeding for a couple more weeks, then decided to bottlefeed. As soon as I switched to bottlefeeding, he started gaining weight! He was quite chubby when I had his picture taken at 3 months. *Judy*

- Until baby begins solids, don't give him extra water unless told to do so by your pediatrician. After he begins eating solids, 1 or 2 ounces of water each day is OK.

Breastfeeding or Bottlefeeding?

- You must decide if you want to breastfeed or bottlefeed your baby. Many people believe that breastfeeding is the best way to feed baby. Breast milk contains every nutrient a baby needs, and it's easily digested.
- Research has found that breastfed babies have lower rates of infection because of the immunological content of breast milk.
- Breastfeeding provides baby a sense of security and mom and dad a sense of self-esteem.

- However, if there are reasons you cannot or choose not to breastfeed your baby, be assured he will do well on formula. It won't harm him if you don't breastfeed.
- An infant can still get all the love, attention and nutrition he needs if breastfeeding is not possible.
- No mother should feel guilty if she doesn't breastfeed her baby.
- We discuss bottlefeeding and breastfeeding in the following sections. See pages 11 and 25.

Feeding More than One Baby

One of the greatest challenges for parents of multiples is deciding how to feed them. Some mothers want to breastfeed exclusively. (It's an added bonus for multiples because they are usually smaller than single-birth babies, and breast milk is extremely beneficial for them.) Some moms say bottlefeeding is the only way to go. Others combine the two, and breastfeed *and* bottlefeed their babies.

- Breastfeeding your babies, even if it's only for one or two feedings a day, gives them the protection from infection that breast milk provides. Research has shown that even the smallest dose of breast milk gives baby an advantage over babies fed only formula.
- One of the best things you can do is to consult a lactation specialist—you're going to need some sound advice. You might want to do this *before* babies are born so you can make a plan.

- If babies are early, and you can't nurse them, begin pumping! Pump from day one, and store your breast milk for the time babies are able to receive it.
- In addition, pumping tells the body to produce breast milk—pump and the milk will come. It just takes some time.
- Breastfeeding multiples is a challenge. If you decide to try it, experiment with various situations and positions to find what works best for you.
- Some mothers nurse both babies at the same time. There are special cushions on the market designed to help you hold and nurse two babies at once.
- Switch babies from one breast to the other at different feedings. This ensures each baby gets visual stimulation on both sides. It also helps prevent problems for you, such as engorgement in one breast if one baby isn't feeding as well as the other. By switching breasts, the demand for milk remains about the same for each breast, so breasts tend to remain equal size.
- Supplementing with formula allows your partner and others to help you feed the babies. You can breastfeed one while someone else bottlefeeds the other.
- Or you can nurse each one for a time, then finish the feeding with formula or pumped breast milk. In either case, someone else can help you feed the babies.
- Be sure to take good care of yourself. Your attempts at breastfeeding may make you feel like a 24-hour fast-food restaurant, but you'll be giving your babies the best start in life.

FROM A MOM'S PERSPECTIVE

My partner pressured me to stop nursing. It became a problem for our intimacy. On the positive side, he liked me having larger breasts. But the nursing pads, breast milk on my clothes and my nursing bra were in his words "a real turn-off." My nursing only lasted 3 weeks. *Barbara*

Try to Get Them on the Same Schedule

- One goal to work toward is getting both babies on the same schedule.
- One baby may be more interested in feeding than the other, but try to feed them both at the same time, when possible.
- Getting your babies to sleep at night at the same time allows you some rest or free time.

Feeding Premature Babies

Breast milk is the best nutrition for a premature baby. It is rich in antibodies and nutrients essential for baby's well-being. However, human milk alone may not provide adequate iron for some premature infants.

- Many preemies are not strong enough to breastfeed, so they are fed electrolyte solutions intravenously (through an I.V.), or they may be fed formula or breast milk through a nasogastric tube that goes into the stomach.

- I.V. solutions contain water, protein, fat, carbohydrates, electrolytes, such as sodium, potassium and chloride, and minerals, such as calcium.
- A premature baby's intestinal system may be too immature to absorb nutrients from milk.
- Feeding through a tube gives your baby the nutrients he needs until he is mature enough to suck and to swallow.
- Baby is fed a small amount at first, but this will gradually be increased as he is better able to handle it.
- As he grows and matures, he learns to suck and to swallow—things that a full-term baby does automatically.
- If a mom can't breastfeed her premature baby, there are specialty formulas available.
- One preemie formula by Enfamil contains DHA and ARA.
- Similac has introduced a formula to use when baby comes home from the hospital.
- Ask your baby's doctor if fortified preemie formula is right for your baby.

Feeding Tips for Trips

Traveling with baby can be an experience—especially if you've never traveled with an infant before! These helpful hints may make feeding your baby during your trip a little more enjoyable.

- One of the most important tips we can give you is *not* to feed baby in a moving car, unless he stays in his car seat. *Never take baby out of his car seat to feed him while the car is moving!*
- If you feed baby formula, refrigerate any prepared formula, if directions call for it.
- If this isn't possible, premeasure water into a clean baby bottle. When baby's hungry, just add powdered formula to the water.
- When possible, bring water from home to mix with formula so it tastes the same.
- You can buy premixed, ready-to-feed formula in cans or bottles. Pour canned formula into a bottle when he's hungry; discard any leftovers.
- It's easy if you breastfeed, as long as you can find a place to feed him where you feel comfortable. Feed baby when he's hungry.
- If you have to be away for a time, pump extra breast milk, then refrigerate or freeze it.

Part II: Bottlefeeding Is One Option

Many women choose to bottlefeed baby. You're not in the minority if you make this choice; studies show that more women bottlefeed than breastfeed. Don't be too hard on yourself or feel guilty if you bottlefeed—it's a personal decision that you are entitled to make. You will *not* be considered a "terrible mother" because you choose not to, or cannot, breastfeed.

Baby will be OK if you choose to bottlefeed. Sometimes a woman cannot breastfeed because of a physical condition or problem. You may be extremely underweight or have some medical condition, such as a prolactin deficiency, heart disease, kidney disease, tuberculosis or HIV. Some infants have problems breastfeeding, or they are unable to breastfeed due to a physical problem, such as a cleft palate or cleft lip. Lactose intolerance can also cause breastfeeding problems.

Some women want to breastfeed and try to, but it doesn't work out. Sometimes you choose not to breastfeed because of other demands on your time, such as a job or other children to care for. Your baby can still get all the love and attention and nutrition she needs if breastfeeding is not possible for you. If breastfeeding doesn't work for you, please don't worry about it. It's OK!

FROM A MOM'S PERSPECTIVE

I really wanted to breastfeed my fourth baby, but I had three other kids to take care of, ages 2½, 4 and 5. There was just so much going on—I couldn't run them all over and still have the time to breastfeed. I tried for a while, but it was too hard. Even now, I feel guilty that I couldn't do it. *Wendy*

Bottlefeeding Is an Individual Choice

Though bottlefeeding is not cheap—you'll spend $1500 to $2000 to feed your baby formula for the first year—we know that through the use of iron-fortified formula, your baby can receive good nutrition if you bottlefeed. Some women also enjoy the freedom bottlefeeding provides. It can make it easier for someone else to help care for the baby. There are other advantages to bottlefeeding.

- You can determine exactly how much formula your baby is taking in at each feeding.
- Bottlefeeding is easy to learn; it never causes you discomfort if it's done incorrectly.
- Fathers can be more involved in caring for baby.
- Bottlefed babies may go longer between feedings because formula is usually digested more slowly than breast milk.
- A day's supply of formula can be mixed at one time, saving time and effort.

- You don't have to be concerned about feeding your baby in front of other people.
- It's easier to bottlefeed if you plan to return to work soon after your baby is born.
- If you feed your baby iron-fortified formula, she won't need iron supplementation.
- If you use fluoridated tap water to mix formula, you may not have to give your baby fluoride supplements.

Bonding with a Bottlefed Baby

Most parents want to establish a strong bond with their baby. However, some parents fear bottlefeeding will not encourage closeness with their child. They fear that bonding will not occur between parent and baby.

- It's not true that a woman must breastfeed her baby to bond with her.
- Formula takes longer to digest than breast milk, so you may not have to feed baby as often.
- However, feeding smaller amounts more frequently helps you bond. It's also easier on baby's immature digestive system.
- There are many ways you can bond with your baby, even if you bottlefeed.
- Studies show that carrying your baby close to your body in a slinglike carrier helps the bonding process. It's great because dads can also bond this way with baby.

- There are other ways you can bottlefeed a baby that can help develop a closer bond between parent and child. Try the following ideas.
  - ~ Find a comfortable place to feed, such as a rocking chair.
  - ~ Snuggle your baby close to you during feeding.
  - ~ Make lots of eye contact, caress her, cuddle her, coo, sing and talk to her.
  - ~ If you feed her warm formula, heat it to body temperature by running a filled bottle under warm water.
  - ~ Rock gently.
  - ~ When she's finished, remove the bottle but continue to hold her close.

What's the Best Way to Bottlefeed Baby?

- Hold the baby in a semi-upright position, with her head higher than her body.
- Place the bottle's nipple right side up, ready to feed; don't touch the tip of the nipple.
- Brush the nipple lightly over the baby's lips, and guide it into her mouth. Don't force it.
- Tilt the bottle so the neck is always filled, keeping the baby from sucking in too much air.
- Remove the bottle during feeding to let baby rest. It usually takes 10 to 15 minutes to finish feeding a bottle.

- Don't leave the baby alone with the bottle. Never prop up a bottle and leave her alone to suck on it.
- Never put a baby down to bed with a bottle.
- There's no evidence that feeding refrigerated formula without warming it will harm your baby. If you usually warm it, your baby will probably prefer it that way.
- If your baby is usually breastfed, she will probably prefer a warmed bottle. Be careful formula is not too hot.

Formulas to Consider

When choosing a formula to feed your baby, there isn't much difference among the brands of regular formula available. Most babies do well on milk-based formula. Formulas are packaged in powder form, concentrated liquid and ready to feed. The end product is the same. All formulas sold in the United States must meet the same minimum health standards set by the Food and Drug Administration (FDA), so they are all nutritionally complete. There are several types of formula on the market today besides regular milk-based formula. They include the following:
- milk-based, lactose-free formula for babies with feeding problems, such as fussiness, gas and diarrhea, that are caused by lactose intolerance
- hypoallergenic protein formula (easier to digest and lactose-free) for babies with colic or other symptoms of milk-protein allergy

- soy-based formula, milk-free and lactose-free for babies with cow's milk allergies or sensitivity to cow's milk

New formulas on the market now include two nutrients found in breast milk—DHA and ARA.

- DHA (docosahexaenoic acid) contributes to baby's eye development.
- ARA (arachidonic acid) is important in baby's brain development.
- DHA and ARA are provided through the placenta before birth and in breast milk after birth.
- These two nutrients are especially good for preemies who missed out on them in the 3rd trimester. Ask your doctor about this type of formula for your baby, especially if she was premature.
- Formulas with DHA and ARA are about 20% more expensive than regular formula.
- The benefit of adding these nutrients to formula will take 5 or 10 years to determine.
- Ask your pediatrician about the type of formula you should feed your baby.
- Some formulas are iron fortified. A baby needs iron for normal growth; a recent study showed that too little iron can lead to mild developmental delays.
- The American Academy of Pediatrics (AAP) recommends that a baby be fed iron-fortified formula for the first year of her life. Feeding for this length of time helps maintain adequate iron intake.
- Some researchers caution parents about using soy-based formula. Recent studies suggest it offers no ben-

efits over cow's-milk formula. They also warn that some of the natural compounds found in soybeans may depress an infant's immune system.

- The AAP recommends soy-based formula *only* for newborns severely allergic to the proteins found in cow's milk (about 3% of all babies).

- If your baby must have a special formula—a prescription or a highly processed commercial brand—check with your insurance company to see if all or part of the cost may be covered.

- Some parents are interested in giving their child organic formulas. The milk used in organic formula comes from cows that were not given growth hormones or antibiotics. The food fed to the cows was also free of pesticides. Organic formula is more expensive, but many parents are willing to pay the extra price.

- Some parents ask about goat's milk in an infant's diet—it was once used with fussy babies because we believed it was easier to digest. We now advise parents *not* to give their baby goat's milk. It has a high concentration of protein, which may make it harder for baby to digest.

Feeding Equipment to Use

- When you feed baby her bottle, use one that is slanted. Research has shown this design keeps the nipple full of milk, which means she takes in less air.

FROM A MOM'S PERSPECTIVE

I wanted to breastfeed all five of my children but had to stop with each one after a few weeks. My OB-GYN said I was losing too much weight breastfeeding, and it wasn't good for my health. *Anne*

- A slanted bottle also helps ensure baby is sitting up to drink. When a baby drinks lying down, milk can pool in the eustachian tube, where it can cause ear infections.
- A new type of nipple allows formula or pumped breast milk to be released at the same rate as breast milk flows during nursing. A twist adjusts the nipple to a flow that is slow, medium or fast. In this way, you can find the flow that works best for your baby. The nipple fits on most bottles. Check your local stores if you are interested.

Bottlefeeding Tips

When you bottlefeed, there are some things you can do to help make the experience healthy and happy for you and your baby.

- Wipe off the top of the formula can (liquid or dry) before you open it.
- Follow the manufacturer's instructions exactly when making up the formula.

- Wash your hands before you prepare formula.
- Thoroughly clean feeding equipment before use.
- Be sure formula expiration dates have not expired.
- If you prepare formula or bottles ahead of time, you can refrigerate them for up to 24 hours.
- A bottle can be warm or cold, but choose one method and stick to it. A baby likes consistency.
- Don't heat formula if it is at room temperature; heat only refrigerated formula.
- Before you heat a bottle, remove the nipple and cap.
- Never microwave glass bottles; they might crack or explode.
- Heat 4-ounce bottles for no longer than 30 seconds in a microwave on high. Heat 8-ounce bottles for no longer than 45 seconds.
- After heating, replace the cap and nipple, and invert the bottle 8 to 10 times. Don't shake it.
- Test the temperature of a heated bottle by dripping a bit on the top of your wrist or the inside of your wrist.
- Throw away any formula left in the bottle.
- Get rid of bottle nipples that are hard or stiff, or those that are extremely soft and gummy feeling.
- Once you find a formula baby likes, use it exclusively.
- If you are adding water to powdered formula, sterilize the water you use until your baby is at least 4 months old or until she starts solids. Do this by boiling it for 1 minute.
- Do *not* assume bottled water is safer than tap water. One study showed that nearly 35% of over 100 brands

of bottled water were contaminated with chemicals or bacteria. If you use bottled water, boil it!

- There is no need to sterilize bottles on a regular basis unless you use well water. In that case, boil bottles and nipples for 5 minutes.
- Always sterilize new bottles, nipples, caps and rings for 5 minutes before using them for the first time.

Other Bottlefeeding Pointers

- Bottlefed babies take from 2 to 5 ounces of formula at a feeding. They feed about every 3 to 4 hours for the first month (6 to 8 times a day). If baby fusses when her bottle is empty, it's OK to give her a little more.
- When baby is older, the number of feedings decreases, but the amount of formula you feed at each feeding increases.
- Burp baby after every feeding to help her get rid of excess air.
- You know baby's getting enough formula if she has six to eight wet diapers a day. She may have one or two bowel movements, too.
- Stools of a bottlefed baby are greener in color than a breastfed baby's and more solid.
- If your baby poops after a feeding, it's caused by the *gastrocolic reflex*. This reflex causes squeezing of the intestines when the stomach is stretched, as with feed-

ing. It is very pronounced in newborns and usually decreases after 2 or 3 months of age.

- If you notice any blood or mucus in baby's stools during these first few weeks, it may be an indication of a milk-protein sensitivity.

- Usually a little blood in the stools and occasional fussiness are the only symptoms. These symptoms disappear when baby is put on a hypoallergenic formula. Discuss the problem with your baby's doctor if she has these symptoms.

- If baby doesn't want a feeding, don't force it. Try again in a couple of hours. However, if she refuses two feedings in a row, contact your pediatrician. Baby may be ill.

- Soon after birth, your bottlefed baby was able to discriminate between sugar water and milk. Later, she will be able to express her distaste for what she is drinking. If she doesn't like what she's drinking, she will turn her head away from the bottle and may refuse to drink.

- At about 6 months of age, a baby may become bored with the bottle.

Salmonella?

As baby gets older and begins to move around and can hold things while she's doing so, different situations may arise. One that may cause a parent some concern is baby drinking formula that is not fresh. Occasionally baby will find a bottle of formula she left someplace and drink it. Can it hurt her? Probably not, especially if the formula has been out only a short while. However, if you don't know how long it's been unrefrigerated, you might be concerned about *salmonella*. Signs that baby is having a problem usually occur between 2 and 72 hours after drinking the formula. Watch for diarrhea and/or vomiting. If these symptoms occur, contact your pediatrician.

- If she drinks well from a cup, she may be ready to give up a few bottles a day, but don't push it.
- Even at this age, a baby needs to suck and may not be ready for weaning. Total weaning from the bottle can wait until she's a year old.

Are Plastic Nipples, Bottles and Pacifiers Safe?

Some concern has been raised recently about the plastic that bottle nipples and pacifiers are made of; some parents wonder if they contain DINP (phthalate), a toxic chemical that used to be in many plastic products.

- A spokesman for the Consumer Product Safety Commission (CPSC) recently stated that no products on the market today contain phthalate.

- Nipples and pacifiers are all made of silicone or latex.
- Those that contained phthalate were removed from the shelves in 1998.
- Some news stories have suggested that clear plastic baby bottles might be unsafe because they contain BPA (bisphenol-A).
- These stories implied that heating a baby bottle could cause BPA to leach into formula or breast milk.
- The FDA has studied the situation and maintains these bottles are safe. Their ongoing research has found no problems with baby-bottle usage and no risk from other food containers that contain BPA.
- If you want to make sure your bottles are OK to use, don't heat them in the microwave.
- Instead, heat formula or breast milk on the stove, then put it in a bottle.
- Using soft plastic liners made of opaque, colored plastic is also safe.

A lot of women breastfeed their babies. It's the healthiest way to feed baby, and it can help create a close bond between mother and child. For many women, it's a wonderful, loving time and often completes the birth experience.

A woman's breast milk provides benefits for the baby, including nutritional development and immunological aspects that can't be duplicated by formula feeding. Breast milk provides species-specific and age-specific nutrition for your baby.

Successful breastfeeding begins at birth. Often baby is awake, alert and ready to learn to suck properly. You can usually begin breastfeeding your baby within an hour (or sooner) after he is born. This provides your baby with *colostrum,* the first milk your breasts produce. Colostrum helps boost baby's immune system. Breast milk comes in 12 to 48 hours after birth.

Breastfeeding helps you, too, because it stimulates the pituitary gland to release oxytocin, the hormone that causes your uterus to contract to help keep bleeding to a minimum. New studies show that oxytocin can also lower blood pressure. You may find you cope a little better with all the stress that comes with being a new mother if you breastfeed.

Whether a woman breastfeeds often depends on what her partner thinks about it. Research has shown that if a woman's partner doesn't want her to breastfeed, she usually doesn't. If this is important to you but not to your partner, explain to him the health benefits for baby. Assure him he'll be able to feed baby expressed breast milk. Often a father will be supportive once he understands how positive breast-feeding is for the entire family.

It's not uncommon for a woman to have some difficulties when she begins breastfeeding. Don't be discouraged if this happens to you. It takes some time to discover what works for you and your baby. In this book, we give you lots of use-ful tips and hints to help make breastfeeding your baby a wonderful, beneficial time for you both!

Benefits of Breastfeeding

- There are many reasons to breastfeed your baby, in-cluding getting close to him, giving him the best nutri-tional start you can and feeling good about how you are taking care of him. There are also benefits for you; see page 33.
- All babies receive from their mother some protection against disease before they are born.
- During pregnancy, antibodies are passed from the mother to the fetus through the placenta. These anti-bodies circulate through the baby's blood for a few months after the baby is born.
- Breastfed babies continue to receive protection in the breast milk they receive.

- Colostrum (the first milk that comes from the breast) that is produced and secreted immediately after birth gives a high level of immune protection.
- The American Academy of Pediatrics (AAP) recommends breastfeeding exclusively for the first 6 months of baby's life.
- Nursing the first 4 weeks of your baby's life provides the most protection for your baby and the most beneficial hormone release to help you recover after the birth.
- Nursing for the first 6 months provides baby excellent nutrition and protection from illness. After 6 months, the nutrition and protection aspects are not as critical for your baby.
- If you can breastfeed only a short period of time, that's OK. Try to stick with it for the first 6 months or at least for the first 4 weeks.

Preventing Infections and Other Health Advantages

- In the first 4 to 7 days after birth, protein and mineral concentrations in breast milk decrease, and water, fat and lactose increase due to baby's changing needs.
- The composition of breast milk continues to change to match baby's nutritional needs. This includes the right balance of immune factors and nutrients. Other factors act as biologic signals for promoting growth of cells.
- Breast milk contains many substances that have antimicrobial properties, which help prevent infection.

- Researchers believe the protein in breast milk helps jump-start baby's immune system.
- Breastfed babies get fewer infections because breast milk is bacteria free and helps a newborn avoid disease. This can mean fewer visits to the doctor and hospital, which can mean you and your partner won't have to miss work to care for a sick baby.
- The incidence of ear infections is significantly reduced (by almost 50%) in babies who breastfeed longer than 4 months.
- Nursing may help prevent diarrhea in infants, and it may inhibit the growth of bacteria that cause urinary-tract infections.
- Baby's permanent teeth may come in straighter if he is breastfed.
- You may lower your baby's chances of developing diabetes if you breastfeed exclusively for the first 2 months of his life.
- Breastfed babies are less likely to develop allergies and asthma. Studies show that babies fed only breast milk for 6 months had fewer instances of asthma, food allergies and eczema into their teen-age years.
- It's nearly impossible for a baby to become allergic to his mother's breast milk, so breastfeeding may prevent milk allergies. This is important if there is a history of allergies in your family or your partner's family. The longer a baby breastfeeds, the less likely he is to be exposed to substances that could cause allergy problems.

FROM A MOM'S PERSPECTIVE

I breastfed *and* bottlefed my baby. She did real well breastfeeding, but my breasts got engorged, and I was too sore and tender to continue. The bottle was a forced decision. *Stephanie*

- Breastfeeding may also lower the risk of a baby developing juvenile diabetes, lymphoma and Crohn's disease later in life.
- Another benefit to breastfeeding is the presence of DHA and ARA in breast milk. DHA (decosahexaenoic acid) is the primary structural fatty acid that makes up the retina of the eye, and ARA is important to development of the gray matter of the brain. During pregnancy, your baby receives these important substances through the placenta. After birth, your breast milk continues to supply them to your baby. Studies have shown that a baby with DHA and ARA in his diet may have a higher IQ and greater visual development than babies fed formula without them.

Other Good Reasons to Breastfeed

- Breast milk is easily digested—for a preemie, it is often the best nourishment.
- When you nurse, breast milk can't get contaminated, be mixed incorrectly or be served at the wrong temperature.

> ### *Will You Lose Weight Breastfeeding?*
>
> Many women have been told they will automatically lose weight if they breastfeed. They falsely believe they don't have to watch what they eat. It does take extra calories to nurse a baby, but the average is only about 500 extra calories a day. If you don't pay attention to what you eat and the quality of calories you take in, it's easy to *gain* weight! So eat nutritiously, keep drinking lots of fluids, exercise and get plenty of rest. You'll soon see the pounds begin to disappear.

- Breastfeeding can save your family money (you don't have to buy formula).
- It's even good for the environment! You don't have to be concerned about disposal of formula cans, bottles and bottle liners.
- Breastfeeding is an excellent way to bond with your baby. Closeness between mother and child can be established during the feeding process.

Disadvantages to Breastfeeding

- Let's be honest—there are some disadvantages to breastfeeding.
- Breastfeeding ties you completely to the baby. Because a woman must be available when her baby is hungry, other family members may feel left out.
- A mother who breastfeeds must also pay careful attention to her diet—what she eats and what she avoids are important. Foods and substances may pass into her

> ### Taking Medication or Drinking a Glass of Wine
>
> If you must take medication for a problem or you want an occasional glass of wine or beer, the best time for you to have these substances is immediately after you finish breastfeeding. Your body will have time to process the medication or alcohol, and it probably won't get into your breast milk in any large quantity.

breast milk and may cause problems for baby. Most substances you eat or drink (or take orally, as medication) can pass to your baby in your breast milk. Spicy foods, cabbage, broccoli, chocolate and caffeine are some things your baby may react to when you eat them.

- A nursing mother shouldn't pump her own gas and should avoid nail polish and exposure to paint fumes. Wait until baby is weaned to get new carpeting, and use cleaning products that are safe for the environment. These substances contain chemicals that could pass into your breast milk.
- Breastfeeding should never feel like a chore—if it does, your baby will be able to sense it.
- If it's not enjoyable to you, you'll be less likely to bond with your baby.

How Breastfeeding Affects You

- After birth, most women's breasts return to their prepregnancy size or decrease a little in size. If you breastfeed, it takes longer for your breasts to return to normal. This is a result of the change in the connective tissue that forms the support system of your breasts.

- Breastfeeding makes even greater demands on your body than pregnancy. You burn about 500 calories a day just to produce milk.
- You may not be getting enough zinc, vitamin D, vitamin E, calcium or folate. Lack of these vitamins and minerals may leave you feeling irritable and tired.
- Ask your doctor about continuing your prenatal vitamins while breastfeeding because they contain what you need.
- You must pay careful attention to your eating plan, both for what you eat and drink and what you should avoid. It's also important to eat particular foods. If you eat these foods while you're breastfeeding, you help your baby obtain these important nutrients.
  - ~ We know choline and docosahexaenoic acid (DHA) can help build baby's brain cells during breastfeeding.
  - ~ Choline is found in milk, eggs, whole-wheat bread and beef.
  - ~ DHA is found in fish, egg yolks, poultry, meat, canola oil, walnuts and wheat germ.
- Research indicates a woman should avoid eating peanuts and peanut products if she breastfeeds. If a child has a predisposition to a peanut allergy, exposure through breast milk as an infant could trigger the allergy, which can be very dangerous in some people.

Do You Smoke?

If you smoke while you breastfeed, be aware that nicotine and its by-product, cotinine, may be found in your breast milk and in your baby's urine. Although researchers are not sure how these substances can affect your baby, it's a good reason to stop smoking. If you can't stop smoking, keep breastfeeding. Breast milk may help protect your baby from some of the unfavorable side effects of secondhand smoke.

Peanut proteins pass into breast milk, and thus to the infant. See the discussion on page 113.

The Benefits of Breastfeeding

- There are many benefits for you if you breastfeed.
- Breastfeeding may help metabolize fat deposits your body laid down during pregnancy.
- It causes hormones to be released that produce uterine contractions and help decrease bleeding. These hormones also help you relax and help you bond with your baby.
- Breastfeeding is linked to a decreased risk of later development of ovarian and breast cancer.
- Breastfeeding delays the onset of menstrual periods following delivery.
- Some studies show a decreased chance of osteoporosis and hip fracture after menopause in women who breastfed their children.

Medications You May Take

As we've already said, most substances you eat or drink can pass to your baby in your breast milk. Keep this in mind when you take prescription *and* over-the-counter medication!

- Be very careful with any medication you take. Although there are many situations in which medication is beneficial for you, sometimes it can have a negative effect on baby.
- Take a medication *only* when you really need it, and take it *only* as prescribed. Ask your physician for the smallest dose possible.
- Check with your pharmacist, your OB-GYN and your pediatrician to see if it's OK to use a particular medication while breastfeeding. Ask about possible effects on the baby, so you can be alert for them.
- Postpone treatment, if possible.
- Consider taking a medication immediately after nursing; it may have less of an effect on the baby.
- If a medication could have serious effects on your baby, you may decide to bottlefeed for the time you must take the medication. You can maintain your milk supply by pumping (then throwing away) your expressed milk.
- Some safe medications to use during breastfeeding include:
  - ~ pseudoephedrine (Sudafed, Actifed)
  - ~ dextromethorphan (Benylin, Robitussin DM)

Do You Take Antidepressants?

If you take antidepressants, your doctor may have advised you not to breastfeed. However, research has shown that some antidepressants are OK to use while nursing. Among mothers taking tricyclic antidepressants, such as *Elavil,* no ill effects have been reported on breastfeeding babies. These drugs have been in use in the United States for over 40 years. There is less information available on newer drugs, such as selective serotonin reuptake inhibitors (SSRIs), which include *Prozac.* However, studies have shown no harm to babies who nursed while their mothers took the drug. Many medical authorities believe that breastfeeding benefits outweigh the possible risks of taking antidepressants. Discuss the situation with your doctor if you have questions.

- ~ acetaminophen (Tylenol), ibuprofen (Alleve)
- ~ attapulgite (Kaopectate)
- ~ topical hydrocortisone (Cortaid)
- ~ calamine lotion, certirizine (Zyrtec)
- ~ loratadine (Claritin)
- ~ intranasal steroid spray (Flonase)
- ~ calcium carbonate (Tums, Maalox)
- ~ codeine
- ~ tetracycline
- ~ amoxicillin
- ~ insulin
- ~ thyroid medications
- ~ prednisone and most antihistamines.
- • Avoid radioactive drugs, anticancer drugs, ergotamine (for migraines), aspirin and lithium.

- Be careful with herbs when you nurse. Avoid comfrey, fennel, sage, ginseng and fenugreek. Fennel and sage used as herbs in cooking are acceptable, if they are used in small quantities.

Birth Control while Breastfeeding?

- While you are breastfeeding, you may not have menstrual periods and you may not ovulate, meaning you won't get pregnant.
- Breastfeeding usually inhibits the production of gonadotropin for an average of 17 weeks. However, be aware that research shows that *80%* of all breastfeeding women ovulate before their first period. About 40 of every 100 women who use breastfeeding for birth control get pregnant!
- Don't rely on breastfeeding alone if you don't want another pregnancy right away. *Take precautions.*
- Be careful with oral contraceptives; hormones can get into your milk and be passed to your baby. Choose some other form of birth control until you are finished breastfeeding.
- You may choose a "minipill" (a progesterone-only birth-control pill), an IUD, Norplant or Depoprovera; all have been proved safe to use if you nurse.
- In addition, new on the scene is *Mirena,* an intrauterine contraceptive (IUD) that can be inserted following delivery, such as at your 6-week checkup. It lasts for 5

years and has proved 99.9% effective. It has the lowest dose of hormones of any of the prescription contraceptives.

- *Implanon* is a flexible plastic implant placed under the skin like Norplant. It releases hormones to prevent pregnancy and has proved 99.9% effective for up to 3 years.
- Barrier methods may also be used; they include condoms, a diaphragm or a cervical cap.

Bonding with a Breastfed Baby

Breastfeeding is an excellent way to bond with your baby because of the physical closeness. Don't be discouraged if breastfeeding doesn't feel natural to you at first. It takes some time to find out what works best for you and your baby.

- Sit in a comfortable chair.
- Hold your baby so he can easily reach the breast while nursing; hold him across your chest or lie in bed.

Some Reasons You May not Be Able to Breastfeed

- You may be unable to breastfeed if you are extremely underweight or have a particular medical condition, such as a prolactin deficiency, heart disease, kidney disease, tuberculosis or HIV.
- Some infants have problems breastfeeding, or they will be unable to breastfeed, if they have a cleft palate or cleft lip.
- Lactose intolerance can also cause breastfeeding problems.

- He should take your nipple into his mouth fully, so his gums cover the areola. He can't suck effectively if your nipple is only slightly drawn into his mouth.
- Look into baby's eyes as he feeds. Sing or talk to him.
- Let him set the pace. For the first few weeks, feed baby 8 to 10 times a day, for 20 to 30 minutes at each feeding. Take more time if your baby needs it.

Is Baby Getting Enough Milk?

You may be concerned about how much breast milk your baby gets at a feeding. There are clues to look for. Watch his jaws and ears while he eats—is he actively sucking? At the end of a feeding, does he fall asleep or settle down easily? Can he go $1^{1}/_{2}$ hours between feedings? You'll know your baby is getting enough to eat if he:

- nurses frequently, such as every 2 to 3 hours or 8 to 12 times in 24 hours
- has six to eight wet diapers and two to five bowel movements a day
- gains 4 to 7 ounces a week or at least 1 pound a month
- appears healthy, has good muscle tone and is alert and active

Some warning signs to be alert for include:

- your breasts show little or no change during pregnancy
- no engorgement after baby's birth
- no breast milk by the 5th postpartum day
- you can't hear baby gulping while he breastfeeds
- your baby loses more than 10% of his birth weight
- baby wets fewer than six diapers and has fewer than two stools a day
- baby never seems satisfied

A baby may get extra hungry at times if he is breastfed exclusively. You may notice periods of extreme hunger in your baby around 10 days, 3 weeks, 6 weeks and 3 months of age. If you have any concerns, discuss them with your baby's doctor or your OB-GYN. To help boost your supply of breast milk, try the following.

- Nurse more often.
- Don't use bottles or pacifiers.
- Express breast milk *after* a feeding; this tells your body to produce more milk.
- Drink lots of water, and eat small meals and protein snacks throughout the day.

Insufficient Milk Syndrome

- Insufficient milk syndrome describes a situation in which baby becomes dehydrated because of breast-feeding problems, such as the mother's low milk supply or the baby's failure to drink enough milk.
- It can happen when a mother has the idea that breast-feeding is the only "right" method of feeding and takes it to extremes.
- This woman views using a bottle as a personal failure, even when breastfeeding complications occur.
- It can also happen when a mother is unable to produce enough breast milk, due to genetic defect, injury or breast surgery.
- What's important to know is that insufficient milk syndrome is rare.
- If you believe you are not producing enough milk or your baby is not getting enough, call your OB-GYN or baby's pediatrician.

Breastfeeding More Than One Baby

If you have more than one baby, you should be able to breastfeed them. You may find it more challenging, but many mothers have done it.

- You may have to be creative in your approach, but with time, you'll probably work it out quite well. You may try to breastfeed exclusively.

- Or you may decide to pump your breasts and divide the breast milk between (or among) your babies, then supplement with formula.
- You may breastfeed your babies for a short while at every feeding, then feed them formula.
- Studies have shown that frequent nursing stimulates milk production.
- Talk with your physician and your pediatrician about what might work best for you and your babies.
- You may also want to consult a lactation specialist.
- Also see the discussion of feeding multiples on page 6.

Other Breastfeeding Facts

- Breast milk becomes more plentiful between 2 and 6 days after baby's birth, when it changes from colostrum to milk.
- Breast milk is easily digested by your baby, so he needs to eat quite often.
- For the first few weeks, feed your baby every 2 to 3 hours around the clock, for 20 to 30 minutes at each feeding. Give baby as much time as he needs to feed.
- It's best to avoid bottles for the first month of breast-feeding for two reasons. Your baby may come to prefer feeding from a bottle (it's not as hard to suck), and your breasts may not produce enough milk.
- If your baby is sick or premature, and you want to breastfeed, pump your breasts and store the milk until

you can feed your baby. This will help establish your milk production, and you'll have a good supply of breast milk on hand when baby comes home.

- If you have enough breast milk stored, you may want to consider donating your extra breast milk to a breast-milk bank. Call your local La Leche League for information.

- Some breastfeeding mothers have special medical problems they must deal with. If you have a chronic illness, you may need to make certain changes in your diet, medication use or daily activities. Discuss the situation with your doctor before making any changes.

- Women who have had breast-enlargement surgery with silicone implants may be able to breastfeed successfully; ask your doctor about it if this concerns you.

- You should also be able to breastfeed after a breast reduction. Milk production may be less after such surgery, but it is usually enough to satisfy the baby.

Milk Letdown

- Many women are surprised when they first experience *milk letdown*.

- Milk letdown is the name for the tingling or cramping a woman feels in her breasts soon after a baby begins to nurse.

- It indicates milk is flowing into breast ducts.

> ### *Do You Need Help with Breastfeeding?*
>
> Breastfeeding can be a challenge—to start and to continue. If you need help with breastfeeding your baby, get it immediately. Ask friends and family members for their advice. Call your doctor's office or your pediatrician—office personnel may be able to refer you to someone knowledgeable, such as a lactation consultant. You can also look in the telephone book for the La Leche League, an organization that promotes breastfeeding. Someone from a local affiliate can give you advice and encouragement. Join a support group; other breastfeeding moms can offer advice and support.

- It occurs several times during feeding; sometimes a baby chokes a bit when the rush of milk comes too quickly.
- You may also experience milk letdown when it's time for your baby to nurse or when you hear a baby crying—your own or any other baby!

Nursing in Public

To date, *more than half* of the states in the United States have passed laws dealing with breastfeeding. Seventeen states have passed laws making it explicitly legal to breastfeed in public. These laws exist to support breastfeeding mothers. In six states, laws have been passed that require employers to give breastfeeding mothers break periods to express milk and a private place in which to do it. In 1999, a federal law was passed that allows women to breastfeed on federal property, including federal office buildings, national parks and museums.

- If you're like most women, you believe nursing your baby is a private time for the two of you.
- However, you may find yourself out and about, with baby screaming at the top of his lungs to be fed *now!*
- Below is a list of some of the places where you can breastfeed baby with some privacy.
  - ~ The women's lounge. This offers some privacy; if someone walks in on you, it's another woman who is probably not offended if you breastfeed your baby.
  - ~ A women's restroom. A lounge may not be available, but a restroom usually is. Go into a stall, close the door and nurse your baby.
  - ~ A fitting room. If baby's crying is getting on everyone's nerves, including your own, dash into a fitting room for a quick feeding.
  - ~ Your car. Park your car in a place that's away from high-traffic areas, and feed baby there.
  - ~ A local park. Your park may have picnic tables and benches that are a little removed from the main area. Using your ever-handy baby blanket, drape it over your shoulder and baby's head for added privacy.
  - ~ Carry baby in a sling. When you carry baby in a front sling designed for breastfeeding, it only takes a minute to undo your nursing top and nursing bra. You can feed baby on the go!

Breastfeeding my baby seemed like it was natural to me. I can't imagine feeding him any other way. I guess we were lucky, to hear stories my friends tell me. My baby latched right on in the delivery room and never had any problems. He grew big, and I breastfed him till he was 10 months old. *Miranda*

Tips to Get Started with Breastfeeding

There are things you can do to help make breastfeeding a success for you both. Below are some things that may help you as you begin nursing.

- Don't be discouraged if you experience difficulty when you first start breastfeeding. It takes some time to work it all out.
- It's not always easy to get started, even though you probably think it's the most natural thing in the world to do.
- It takes practice! Although breastfeeding is a natural way to feed baby, it takes time and practice to get the hang of it.
- Wear the right clothes. Clothes made for nursing help you feel more comfortable; buy nursing bras and tops that let you feed baby without baring all.
- Relax in a comfortable place before you start. Make it a peaceful experience.

- Make sure baby is comfortable. Be sure he's dry and warm.
- Help baby connect with your breast. Brush your nipple across his lips. When he opens his mouth, place the nipple and as much of the areola in his mouth as you can.
- You should feel him pull the breast while sucking, with no pain. If you experience pain, disengage him by slipping your finger into the corner of his mouth and gently pulling down to break the suction.
- Don't rush—it takes time for your baby to nurse, sometimes as long as 25 to 30 minutes.
- Hold your baby so he can reach the breast easily while nursing. His chest should face you, not the ceiling. A straight line should run from his head to his hip. This allows him to latch on better, so your nipples won't get sore.
- Your own position is also important. If you sit up, put a pillow on your lap for arm support as you hold baby. Don't bend over to feed him. He should be on his side, directly in front of you. Placing your feet on a footstool can help relieve pressure on your back.
- If you lie down, have baby's chest facing you, and keep the line straight from his head to his hip.
- Your baby should take your nipple fully into his mouth, so his gums cover the areola. He can't suck effectively if your nipple is only slightly drawn into his mouth.
- Nurse baby 5 to 10 minutes on each breast; he gets most of his milk at the beginning of the feeding.

- Add some cover. A receiving blanket helps add privacy to your nursing experience.
- A breastfed baby may not need burping. As you begin, burp between feeding at each breast and when baby finishes. If he doesn't burp, don't force it. He may not need to burp.
- If you see a blister on baby's lip, it is probably from sucking. It isn't painful, and you don't have to do anything for it. It'll disappear on its own.
- Between 6 weeks and 6 months, baby grows quickly. He will probably take in about 3 to 4 ounces of milk each day for every pound of weight during this time.
- Work around baby's feeding schedule. As he gets older, you'll be in tune with his schedule and you can plan your own time more easily.

Breastfeeding Fast Facts

Baby's Feeding Pattern

- You may be unprepared for how often your baby will want (and need) to nurse in the first few weeks after birth.
- Feed your newborn when he's hungry. A baby usually cuts back to 4 to 6 times a day by the age of 4 months.
- You may wonder if it's worth it to continue. Relax and be patient.
- It takes time for your baby to establish his nursing pattern.

- By the end of the 2nd or 3rd week, a pattern will probably become established, and your baby will sleep longer between feedings.

FROM A MOM'S PERSPECTIVE

My husband, Jeff, was jealous. He resented the time I spent cuddling the baby. It was hard because I loved the private moments with our beautiful daughter, even in the middle of the night. Jeff had had similar feelings of being left out during the pregnancy, and it had created tension between us. We talked about why I should breastfeed, and he finally saw the light. It was good to work out our problems together. It made our relationship stronger, and we grew together as a family. *Marti*

Avoid Bottles when Possible

- It's best to avoid bottles to supplement breastfeeding for the first month of breastfeeding if you can.
- Your baby may come to prefer feeding from a bottle (it's not as hard to suck).
- Your breasts may not produce enough milk.

What Is Nipple Confusion?

- *Nipple confusion* refers to a baby's confusion about sucking on a rubber nipple and sucking on his mother's breast.

- About 25% of all breastfed babies who receive a bottle during the first few weeks after birth have this problem.
- Different mouth and tongue movements are required to suck on a breast than to suck on a rubber nipple.
- Alternating between breast and bottle can lead to sucking problems (confusion).
- For this reason, don't offer baby a bottle or pacifier until he is 6 to 8 weeks old.

Breastfeeding at Work or while You're Away

- It is possible to continue breastfeeding your baby after you return to work.
- If you breastfeed exclusively, you will have to pump your breasts or arrange to see your baby during the day.
- Or you can nurse your baby at home and provide formula when you're away.
- You may find it necessary to be away from your baby for a few days during breastfeeding. If this is necessary, you will probably need to pump your breast milk while you are gone.
- If you don't, you may be very uncomfortable because breast milk will continue to come in. Take a breast pump with you, and discard the breast milk after it is pumped.

Your Away-from-Home Breastfeeding Kit

If you need to be away from baby—for work or for some other reason—and you want to pump your breasts, it's a good idea to have some essentials with you. Put them all together in a small bag, and you'll be all set, no matter where you are. Include in your kit the items listed below:

- a good breast pump
- storage containers or bags for the breast milk
- some no-water antibacterial hand cleaner, in case you can't wash your hands
- nipple cream
- nipple shields or pads
- some extra clothes, including a couple of nursing bras and a neutral-colored blouse, in case you have any leaks

Clothes to Wear while Breastfeeding

- It may be most comfortable to wear a nursing bra if you breastfeed. Nursing bras have cups that open so you can breastfeed without having to get undressed. They also provide very good support for your enlarged breasts. You may want to wear one 24 hours a day, even when you sleep at night.
- There are other special clothes you might want to consider wearing if you breastfeed. Many nightgowns, shift dresses and full-cut blouses have discreet breast openings so you don't have to get undressed to breastfeed. You can reach up inside your outer clothing, un-

hook your nursing bra and place your baby at your breast without anyone noticing.

- Lightly draping a towel or baby blanket over your shoulder and over the baby's head adds further coverage.
- A "nursing cape" can be used to provide privacy. The cape is a large square of fabric, with a head-sized opening in the middle. The hole is placed over the mother's head, and the rest of the fabric covers the mother's chest and back, also covering the nursing baby. No blankets to slip off your shoulder!

Can Others in the Family Help Feed Baby?

- You can help make your partner feel he is part of the family when you breastfeed.
- He can help out by getting up at night and bringing the baby to you or by changing the baby.
- Your partner can also feed your baby expressed breast milk.
- You can include other family members, such as older children, by letting them hold or burp the baby after he is fed.
- If you express your milk, an older child could feed the baby a bottle of it at a feeding.

Switching Breasts during Breastfeeding

- It's a good idea to switch breasts during breastfeeding. You can wait until your baby finishes with one breast

FROM A MOM'S PERSPECTIVE

Everybody told me breastfeeding was good for me and my baby. But they didn't tell me how tied down I'd be. I couldn't go anywhere or do much of anything while I was breastfeeding. I decided to stop when I realized how much I missed my friends. After I started bottlefeeding, I could go out dancing and have fun again! *Bev*

before switching to the other one. Or you may want to switch after 10 or 15 minutes of nursing.

- At the next feeding, start your baby on the breast you nursed last. This helps you keep both breasts stimulated and producing milk.
- If your baby only wants to nurse from one breast each feeding, switch to the other breast the next feeding.
- If baby only wants to nurse on one breast, such as the right breast, at every feeding, making some changes may help. Try a different place to feed him, such as using a chair when you've been feeding him lying down, or change the way you hold him.

How Baby Handles Breastfeeding

- After you get into the routine of breastfeeding, baby will settle into a feeding schedule.

- He will feed as often as he needs to. You may notice as he gets older that he will drop a feeding but increase the amount he takes in at each feeding.
- Your milk supply will be well established.
- If your doctor is concerned about baby's development, he or she will discuss it with you at your next well-baby check.

When Baby Spits Up

- It's not unusual for a baby to spit up after a feeding, especially for a newborn.
- *Spitting up* is not a cause for worry—baby is getting rid of excess breast milk or formula.
- As he spends more time sitting up, he'll outgrow this. Most babies outgrow spitting up by 8 to 12 months of age.
- Until he gets older, keep a cloth handy to wipe up any baby spit-up.
- *Vomiting* occurs when a baby forcibly ejects stomach contents, usually in large amounts.
- Nearly every baby vomits occasionally, and for many different reasons. If your baby vomits more often, contact your doctor.

Burping Baby

- Some breastfed babies don't need to be burped. Some do. Bottlefed babies do need to be burped.

- But how do you burp a baby?
- There are three techniques to use when burping a baby.
- Try them all, and use what works best for your baby.
- Whichever way you hold him, rub or gently pat his back until he burps.
  - ~ Hold baby seated in your lap, with his head in one of your hands.
  - ~ Hold him facing you in your arms, against your chest.
  - ~ Lay him face down on your lap, supporting his head with your hand.

Supplemental Feedings

- If you must provide your baby with supplemental feedings while you breastfeed, wait until you've been breastfeeding for at least 4 weeks, if possible.
- This gives your body a chance to adjust and ensures a good milk supply.
- It also keeps baby from taking a liking to a bottle (it's much easier to feed).
- Some babies refuse to breastfeed after they become used to a bottle.
- Occasional supplemental feedings shouldn't be a problem after 4 weeks.

Vitamin Supplements

- If your baby was full-term, he probably won't need too many vitamin supplements.

- Premature infants may need additional iron because they didn't store it up before birth. Discuss it with your pediatrician if you are concerned.
- In some special situations, vitamins may be recommended. This is a decision for your doctor to make. Do *not* give your baby any supplements without discussing it first with your pediatrician.
- Most doctors suggest *you* continue taking prenatal vitamins.
- Don't take extra vitamins, minerals or herbs unless your doctor tells you to do so.
- The AAP recommends that *all* babies from the age of 2 months (continuing until baby is drinking 17 ounces a day of vitamin-D fortified milk) receive 200IU of vitamin D every day to prevent rickets.
- Vitamin-D supplements alone are very concentrated and unsafe to use for children. The AAP recommends using a multivitamin containing 200IU of vitamin D, which is available over the counter in tablets or liquid form.
- In the past, parents were advised to put a baby outside in the sunshine because he needed vitamin D. The baby got vitamin D from the sun's ultraviolet rays. Dr. Benjamin Spock's baby book actually included a schedule for "sunbathing baby." Parents were also advised that baby needed lots of fresh air. Many babies spent as long as 2 or more hours a day outside, but thankfully only a short time in direct sunlight! We don't recommend this practice today! Talk to your

baby's doctor if you have questions or are confused about vitamin-D supplementation.

- Fluoride helps the development of baby's healthy teeth. Discuss with your pediatrician your baby's need for a fluoride supplement. Most pediatricians begin fluoride supplementation when a baby is about 6 months old. Correct dosage is based on the amount of fluoride in your water supply and whether your baby is receiving any of that water.

- Use of powdered formula, made with local water, compared to ready-to-use formula or breast milk, may determine if your baby needs supplementation.

- Too much fluoride can result in discolored or mottled teeth, so follow your pediatrician's recommendation.

Baby's Bowels

- Pay attention to baby's bowel movements. A change can alert you to a problem.

- Your breastfed baby's bowel movements may become more infrequent as he grows older. He may poop only once every few days.

- If the amount of baby's stool—too much, too little— changes, or the stool differs from your child's normal pattern, you may want to call baby's doctor.

- If any change in baby's stool is associated with a decrease in appetite or fussiness, contact your pediatrician.

- If you notice any blood in the stool, call your doctor or take baby to the emergency room.

- The most common cause of blood in the stool is an anal fissure, which is a tiny cut or tear in the anal opening.

Some Warning Signs for You and Baby

You need to take extra-special care of yourself when you breast-feed. Below are signs that might indicate you have a problem. If you experience any of these problems, call your doctor immediately:

- fever or chills
- extreme fatigue and body aches, as if you have the flu
- burning pain in either or both breasts
- red streaks on the breast
- lumpy areas in your breasts
- feeling of warmth in either breast
- swollen breasts, which keep baby from latching onto the nipple
- sore, cracked or bleeding nipples
- milk that does not flow freely
- low milk supply
- any feelings of depression or extreme sadness

Warning signs may also be seen in your baby. Call your pediatrician if baby:

- doesn't wake up or doesn't stay awake long enough to nurse
- is fussy after nursing and cannot be settled by feeding again
- wets fewer than 6 diapers a day
- has fewer than 2 bowel movements a day
- has signs of jaundice

Pumping and Storing Your Breast Milk

There may be times you need to be away from baby but still supply him with breast milk to drink. With the great array of gadgets available today, it's easy to supply your baby with the breast milk he needs.

- To have breast milk available so baby can drink it while you're away from him, you can "express" it. Do this by using a breast pump (hand, battery or electrically operated) to remove milk from your breasts. Expressed milk can be refrigerated or frozen and saved.
- Milk doesn't need immediate refrigeration; it will stay fresh up to 4 hours at temperatures as high as 77F and 24 hours at 60F.
- It takes time to express your milk. You'll need 10 to 30 minutes to do it, depending on the type of pump you have. Electric pumps work the best. You can buy one, or you may be able to rent one at a medical supply store.
- You'll probably have to express your milk 1 to 4 times a day (around the time you would normally nurse).
- Find a comfortable, private place where you can relax enough for milk letdown to occur.
- Don't bottlefeed your baby with formula, if you have a choice. Your milk supply is driven by your baby's demand.

Storing Breast Milk

Store your breast milk after you express it. There are several steps to take to store breast milk safely.

- Pump or express milk into a clean container.
- Label the container with the date and amount of milk collected.
- You can keep fresh breast milk at room temperature for a few hours; it's best to refrigerate it as soon as possible.
- Breast milk can be safely stored in the refrigerator for up to 72 hours.

Freezing Breast Milk

You can freeze breast milk if you do it properly.

- Use a disposable polyethylene bottle bag or a plastic storage container. If you use bags, double bag the milk for extra protection.
- Mark each container with the amount of milk and the date it was expressed.
- Freeze milk in small portions, such as 2 to 4 ounces, because these amounts thaw more quickly.
- Fill the container only 3/4 full to allow for expansion during freezing.
- You can combine fresh breast milk with frozen breast milk. First, cool *fresh* breast milk (that you have just expressed) before combining it with *thawed* frozen milk. The amount of thawed breast milk must be more than

the amount of fresh breast milk. Never refreeze breast milk!

- In addition, never add fresh, warm milk to already frozen milk.
- There are ways to thaw breast milk so it maintains its high quality.
  - ~ Move the milk from the freezer to the refrigerator; leave for 12 hours.
  - ~ Or you can leave the milk on the counter at room temperature until it thaws.
  - ~ Put the container of frozen milk in a bowl of warm water for 30 minutes, or hold the frozen container under warm running water.
  - ~ **Do not microwave breast milk; it can alter its composition.**
- Swirl the container to blend any fat that might have separated during thawing.
- Feed thawed milk immediately, or store in the refrigerator for up to 24 hours.
- Keep it in a refrigerator freezer for 6 months or in a deep freezer (–20F) for up to 12 months.
- Place milk in the coldest part of the freezer—the back is usually coldest.

Some Common Problems during Breastfeeding

- Your body needs time to adjust to the demands of breastfeeding.

I was only 17 when my little girl was born. I was so scared I'd do something wrong that I decided to bottlefeed her. When my son was born, I was older and did everything right. I breastfed him till he was almost a year old. It's funny how being older helped me be a better mom. *Martha*

- Your nipples need to toughen up before breastfeeding is completely painless.
- However, if you continue to experience pain, or if your nipples bleed or crack, call your doctor. He or she will give you advice.
- Soon after your baby begins to nurse, you will experience a tingling or cramping in your breasts, which means milk is flowing into the breast ducts.
- This is milk letdown and occurs several times during feeding.

Engorgement

- Several days after baby's birth, your milk will change from colostrum to mature milk.
- At that time, your breasts may feel full and hard; this is called *engorgement.* Your breasts may be painful for 24 to 36 hours.
- It's important to continue breastfeeding during this time, even if your breasts are sore.

- To help relieve the soreness, try the following tips.
  - ~ Encourage baby to feed at least every 2 hours, day and night, so within a few days your body can tell how much milk baby actually needs.
  - ~ Use a pump to express about an ounce of breast milk *before* you nurse. This may make baby's latching on easier and less painful because breasts won't be so hard. It also brings milk to the nipple, ready for baby.
  - ~ Wear a bra that offers good support for breasts, and apply cold compresses to your breasts for short periods.
  - ~ A warm shower stimulates milk letdown; this can help with engorgement.
  - ~ Take acetaminophen if pain is severe, but don't take anything stronger, unless your doctor prescribes it.

Sore Nipples

- Your nipples may become sore when you begin breast-feeding.
- One cause may be that baby is latching onto the nipple for longer than necessary.
- When that happens, enzymes in his saliva eat away at the outer layer of the nipple, exposing sensitive tissue.
- Creams and gel pads are available to help deal with the problem.
- If your baby doesn't take your nipple fully into his mouth during breastfeeding, his jaws can compress the nipple and make it sore.

- Sore nipples rarely last longer than a couple of days. It's important to try to continue breastfeeding, even if your nipples are sore.
- There are other ways to help avoid sore nipples.
  - ~ Nipple shields, worn inside your bra between the nipple and bra fabric, provide some relief. They prevent tender skin from rubbing on the bra fabric.
  - ~ A mild cream can also provide soothing relief. Ask your pharmacist or doctor to recommend products that are OK to use during nursing.

Breast Infections (Mastitis)

- You can get a breast infection, also called *mastitis,* while you breastfeed.
- When this happens, you'll likely have one or more of the following symptoms.
  - ~ large red streaks that extend up the breast toward the armpit
  - ~ hard and painful lumps in the breast
  - ~ fever or flulike symptoms
- If you experience any of these symptoms, call your doctor immediately.
- An infection can cause a fever to develop within 4 to 8 hours after the appearance of the red streaks.
- Prompt medical treatment can improve the symptoms and even clear up the infection within 24 hours.
- There are several things you can do if you think you have an infection.

~ Apply a warm compress to the affected area, or soak the breast in warm water.

~ Express milk or breastfeed while massaging the tender area.

~ If you develop flulike symptoms with a sore breast, call your doctor. Antibiotic treatment may be started, but it must be started as soon as possible.

~ You may need to rest in bed.

~ Empty your infected breast by pumping or breastfeeding every hour or two.

~ Left untreated, a breast infection can turn into an abscess. This is very painful and may need to be opened and drained.

• There are several things you can do to help prevent a breast infection.

~ Eat right, and get plenty of rest to keep your immune system working efficiently.

~ Don't wear tight-fitting bras, especially underwire types, because they can block milk flow, which may cause an infection.

~ Empty breasts—through breastfeeding or pumping—on a regular schedule to avoid engorgement.

~ After each feeding or pumping, let nipples air dry for a few minutes.

~ Don't stop nursing if you get a breast infection; it won't harm baby or affect your milk. If you stop, the infection may get worse because you are still making milk. Breasts become more engorged and more painful.

I bottlefed my babies because neither of them was receptive to breastfeeding. *Allie*

Plugged Milk Ducts

- Another situation you might encounter during breast-feeding is a plugged milk duct, which prevents milk from flowing freely.
- A plugged duct is not red and you will not have a fever, but a plugged duct results in areas of the breast that become more painful after breastfeeding.
- Treatment is usually unnecessary with a plugged duct.
- It usually takes care of itself if you continue to nurse frequently.
- Apply warm compresses to the sore area to help with the pain and to help open the duct.
- Acetaminophen may be used for pain.

Colds and Viruses

- If you have a cold or other virus, it's all right to breast-feed.
- If you need to take a medication, ask your doctor or pharmacist if it's OK to use it while breastfeeding.
- Be sure to ask *before* you begin taking any medication.

Introducing the Bottle to a Breastfed Baby

If you find it necessary to feed your breastfed baby from a bottle, there are some things to keep in mind as you help him learn this new skill. It may take some time and repeated effort on your part, but you can help baby by using the techniques described below.

- Don't offer a bottle or pacifier until breastfeeding is well established. Wait as long as you can, at least until 4 weeks, before offering baby a bottle. Introducing one too soon can cause nipple confusion and interfere with your milk supply.
- Let someone else give the baby a bottle. He associates breastfeeding and breast milk with you.
- Offer the first bottle when he's not hungry. If you wait until he's starving, he may be too distressed to eat. If you feed him a bottle when he's only a little hungry, he'll be able to deal with it better.
- Introduce the bottle slowly. Drop a little milk on his lips from the bottle, then wait until he opens his mouth before you put the bottle in.
- Your baby may take to the bottle better if you hold him in a different position than when you nurse him. When bottlefeeding, sit baby in a more upright position.
- Be patient. You may need to try this new feeding method more than once before baby takes to it. If he

gets frustrated, angry or upset, you may need to take a break and try again later.

- A young baby needs to drink from a bottle—don't try to start him on a cup too early. Younger babies have a strong urge to suck, which you must satisfy. And a young baby doesn't have the coordination to get enough fluid from a cup.

- At 6 months, you can begin letting him drink once in awhile from a cup.

From Breast to Bottle

You may decide you want to wean baby from breastfeeding and start him on formula. Below are some tips.

- It's best to *ease* a breastfed baby into formula when you make the switch. Don't do it all at once, or baby may refuse to cooperate.

- Many breastfed babies don't like the taste of formula. To make the change, give him a bottle that contains only 1/4 formula. Express your breast milk, then mix one part formula to three parts breast milk. This allows him to become accustomed to the different taste. Every few days, replace a little more of the breast milk with formula.

- If he refuses to take the bottle when you change the ratio of formula to breast milk, go back to the ratio you were using before. Offer him this for a few days, then add a little more formula while cutting down on the breast milk. Keep it less than the amount he refused.

- Be patient; some babies can take weeks to accept straight formula.
- If your baby has difficulty drinking from a bottle, or refuses to drink from one, you may have to take additional measures.
  ~ He may be able to begin drinking from a cup. This might be a good solution if you can't get him to take his formula mix from the bottle.
  ~ If your baby is 9 months or older, using a cup instead of a bottle is probably the best idea. You won't have to wean him off a bottle in the near future.

Discontinuing Breastfeeding

When you decide to discontinue nursing, you can either taper off gradually or stop "cold turkey." Each way has its advantages.

- If you want to taper off gradually, offer a bottle at every other feeding, or offer bottles during the day and nurse only at night.
- In the past, medication was given to women to stop milk production; however, these medications are no longer used.
- If you stop "cold turkey," you may have some sleepless nights with a screaming baby, and you may be quite

uncomfortable physically with engorged breasts. However, this method takes less time.

- A third method is to let your child set the pace. Nurse baby when he's interested, but don't offer it to him if he isn't.
- Some women like to nurse until they return to work. Others nurse through the first year. It depends on your situation and your desire, and when your baby gets teeth!

Part IV: Beyond the Breast and Bottle— It's Time to Feed Baby Solids

One of the most exciting, and sometimes frustrating, times during your baby's first year is when you begin feeding her solids. Together you will move from baby cereal to vegetables and fruit to finger foods. You'll begin by feeding her, and by the end of her first year, she'll be trying (and often succeeding!) to feed herself.

Eating solid foods—anything beyond breast milk or formula—is an important step forward for baby. She must be ready for the task. You don't want to start too early, and you don't want to wait too long. Together with your pediatrician, you will decide when to begin and how.

We cover the information in this section in chronological order. By that we mean that at the beginning of this section, you'll find information on beginning to feed solid food to baby. Later in the section, we provide information on feeding baby at 6 months, 8 months, 9 months until the end of her first year.

Is Baby Ready for Solid Food?

When your baby turns 4 months, you may be wondering if she is ready to start eating solid food. Every baby is different. Some babies may be ready to start eating solids before other babies of the same age. Following are some things to keep in mind.

- Solid food will *not* make baby sleep through the night, so don't make the decision to feed her solids because you want her to sleep longer.
- If you begin feeding her solids before she's ready, you can actually cause her more problems.
- A baby's digestive system isn't ready for solid food when she's very young. In fact, she'll be about 9 months old before she develops digestive enzymes that help her get the most nutritive value from the foods she eats. However, eating solids is important for baby. She needs to learn how to eat and to experience different food tastes and textures.
- Discuss it with your pediatrician before you make *any* changes in baby's diet.
- Before she can begin eating solid foods, your baby needs to be able to control her head and neck muscles.
- She also needs to be able to move her tongue back and forth.
- These two skills help her avoid choking.
- Most babies do not achieve these skills until they are between 4 and 6 months old.
- Before this age, your baby's *tongue-thrust reflex* is still very strong. This reflex helps baby draw a nipple into her mouth but pushes out solid food.
- The reflex begins to diminish around 4 months, when baby will be better able to take food from a spoon and swallow it.

- Beginning solid foods is a big step in baby's life.
- Below is a checklist to help determine if your baby is ready for this important step. Most, if not all, of the following should apply to baby:
  - ~ controls her neck
  - ~ sits up with support
  - ~ has nearly doubled her birth weight
  - ~ shows when she is full (turns her head or refuses to open her mouth)
  - ~ shows interest in food when you eat
  - ~ mimics you when you eat, such as opening her mouth when you open yours to take a bite
  - ~ indicates her wants by reaching or leaning toward something
  - ~ seems hungry for more food

Beginning Solids—
An Exciting Time for You All

What Food to Feed Baby

- Most pediatricians recommend you start baby on rice or oat cereal made especially for young babies.
- Dry cereals in a box have more iron than jarred baby cereal.
- You can mix the dry cereal with breast milk or formula.
- For her first meals, make cereal very thin, then thicken it as baby gets used to it.

FROM A MOM'S PERSPECTIVE

My baby absolutely refused to nurse on my left breast, no matter what I did! He was so stubborn, and I didn't want to make it unpleasant when I fed him. After 2 months, I noticed my left breast was quite a bit smaller than the right one, so I stopped breastfeeding. After a few months of bottlefeeding, my breasts were once again the same size—still small, but the same size! *Heather*

- If you breastfeed baby, another food you can begin with is mashed bananas. They are sweet, like breast milk, and are less likely to cause food allergies.
- When you start feeding solids, keep giving your baby breast milk or formula.
- Cereal is only a small portion of her diet—2 or 3 *teaspoons* to begin with.
- Discuss with your pediatrician the amount of formula or breast milk and the amount of solids to feed your baby.
- When she is eating well, and you begin to add more variety to her diet, do *not* reduce the amount of fat she consumes.
- Some parents mistakenly believe that reducing fat will keep baby from gaining too much weight.
- However, studies show that fat and protein are crucial for tissue growth and brain development in the first 2 years of life.
- Your baby needs fat in her diet.

How to Begin Feeding Solids to Baby

- You may be wondering how to start the process of feeding baby her first solid food.
- One good idea is to begin by using your finger as her first spoon.
- Wash your hands well, then dip your finger into prepared cereal.
- When she opens her mouth to eat, place a few drops on her lips. Let her suck on your finger.
- Next, place some cereal on the tip of baby's tongue. When she swallows this bit of cereal, place some in the middle of her tongue.
- If she makes faces, it's only her reaction to this new experience.
- Watch her closely to see how she responds to eating solids.
- She may open her mouth wide for more.
- If the food comes back out, it doesn't mean she doesn't like it. She may need to learn to keep her mouth closed to keep the food inside.
- If baby rejects the food, her tongue-thrust reflex may still be strong. Let her practice.
- If she still has trouble, you may need to wait 1 or 2 weeks before trying again.
- As baby becomes more adept at eating cereal, gradually increase the amount she takes in. About 1/4 cup should be sufficient for a meal.

- Feed her solids once a day. Within a month or so, they'll become a regular part of her meals.
- Once you begin, offer her only one new item at a time, and offer it for a while.
- This gives her the chance to become familiar with eating food. It also lets her become familiar with many different tastes.
- If she has an allergic reaction to any of the foods she eats, it's also easier to identify the problem food.

The Logistics of Feeding Baby Solid Food

- When you feed your baby solids, she must be in a sitting position.
- Place her in your lap or her infant seat. As she gets older and sits more confidently, you can place her in a high chair.
- Use a baby spoon or some other small spoon. Her mouth isn't very large, so she won't eat comfortably from a larger spoon.
- There are products available now that tell you if baby's food is too hot. One spoon turns a different color if the temperature of the food is hot.

Be Patient and Take Your Time

- Your baby will take her own time to settle into an eating routine.

- She may eat a couple of tablespoons of cereal one day, then not eat for the next day or two.
- She may like a food one day, then not eat the same food the next.
- Remain calm and reassuring as you begin this new adventure.
- Never try to force her to eat something she doesn't like.
- Wait awhile, then try again. She may like a food the next time.
- Be careful with your own reactions. If you don't like a particular food, baby may sense it and refuse to eat it.

Will Baby Stop Formula or Breast Milk?

- As your baby begins solids, she'll be exposed to a variety of new tastes.
- As she settles into eating solids as a part of her daily diet, she may want to nurse less or drink less formula.
- However, during the first year, breast milk and formula should be the main source of her nutrition.
- Encourage her to keep nursing or taking formula. These are the most complete sources of nutrition, vitamins, minerals and other important substances your baby needs.

Formula or Breast Milk and Solids

- Once your baby begins eating solids on a regular basis, she may be less interested in breast milk or formula,

A Word of Caution

You may have heard from someone, such as your mother or mother-in-law, that putting cereal in a baby's bottle is a good way to start solids. *Don't do it!* When your baby begins solids, it's a new learning experience for her. She needs to develop the techniques for eating solid foods.

but it should continue to be her primary source of protein and calories for her first year.

- Even at 1 year old, about *half* of baby's caloric needs are provided by breast milk or formula.
- Before baby began eating solids, she was drinking between 35 and 40 ounces each day. Over the next few months, her interest in food increases and her interest in nursing or bottlefeeding decreases.
- However, she should still be drinking a little over 20 ounces of breast milk or formula at age 1.

The Scoop on Baby Cereals

You'll have a lot to choose from when you buy baby cereal. There are many to check out before you make your decision. Below are some points to keep in mind as you choose and then begin feeding cereal to baby.

- Begin with rice cereal. This type of cereal causes the fewest food-allergy problems.
- Buy only iron-fortified cereal. Baby needs iron in her diet.

- In the beginning, buy single-ingredient cereal, such as rice, barley or oatmeal. As baby gets used to eating different foods, and has no reactions to them, you can add foods to her cereal or choose cereals that include other foods.
- Begin with a thin mixture—mix 1 teaspoon of cereal with 4 teaspoons of breast milk or formula.
- Don't make more than a small amount because it can go to waste.
- If your baby has any problems eating cereal, call your pediatrician before offering it to her again.
- After baby learns how to move food to the back of her throat and swallow it, you can make the cereal thicker.
- Offer baby cereal once a day, either at breakfast or dinner.
- As she becomes more adept at eating, offer her two "meals" a day, one at breakfast and one at lunch or dinner.
- Feed your baby only one new food a week. In the beginning, this will be one cereal each week.
- As she gets older, you can add different types of baby food, such as fruits and vegetables.
- Discuss it with your pediatrician.

Should You Wait to Introduce Solids?

- There are advantages to starting baby on solid food between 4 and 6 months, so don't postpone it beyond 6 months of age.

- Studies show offering solids before 3 months or after 6 months of age increases your baby's chance of developing Type-1 diabetes.
- Offering baby solid food between 4 and 6 months exposes her to the tastes and textures of a variety of foods.
- Once your baby reaches 9 months, she might have difficulty accepting solids if she hasn't already experienced them.
- Some children gag and have trouble swallowing if they are not offered food until they are older. When this happens, it is hard to overcome the problem.
- She needs experience eating different foods to become proficient at it. It may take her awhile to get the knack, but she soon will.
- Your baby will enjoy the new foods once she's used to them.
- She'll be more satisfied, too, because solids fill her up more than formula or breast milk.

Tips for Feeding Baby

Embarking on this new experience with baby can be fun *and* frustrating. It's exciting to see her begin to eat food; she's growing up! Soon she may be part of the family during mealtimes. It can also be frustrating to feed her because this new activity can take some time to master. Keep your cool when you feed her, and keep in mind the following suggestions.

- When she can sit up well, put her in a high chair to feed her. It's more convenient for you and more fun for her.
- When you warm her food, don't make it too hot. Always stir her food well, and taste it before you feed it to her. Her mouth is sensitive to hot food, and you could easily burn her tongue.
- Don't add anything to baby's food, such as salt, sugar, pepper or any other flavoring. Avoid honey at all costs! See the discussion on page 103.
- Use a small spoon to feed her. She has a small mouth, so a regular-sized spoon is too big and could cause problems, such as too much food or difficulty getting the spoon in and out of her mouth.
- Don't put food in her bottle. She needs to learn to eat it, not drink it!
- Keep trying. It can take some time for baby to learn all she needs to know to eat solids. It'll be awhile before she settles into eating solid foods.

She May Need to Suck More

- You may be surprised if your baby displays the need to suck more.
- This may occur as baby sucks less on the breast or bottle because she is now eating solid food.
- Baby may also be frustrated by her attempts at locomotion and be trying to soothe herself.
- She may need a pacifier to satisfy her desire to suck.

FROM A MOM'S PERSPECTIVE

I loved breastfeeding my kids. I did it the longest with my first baby. I decided to stop breastfeeding him when he was old enough to ask for it! *Helen*

Packing Your Diaper Bag

Now that solids are a part of your baby's daily diet, you may need to make some adjustments and/or additions in what you pack when you go out. Below are some ideas we've gathered for you.

- Put a premeasured amount of dry cereal in a zipping plastic bag. Or buy dry cereal in premeasured packets. These are convenient to carry with you.
- Put a premeasured amount of dry cereal in a plastic bowl with a lid. When you want to feed baby, just add breast milk or formula.
- To make it even simpler, if you bottlefeed, add dry formula (in the correct amount) to the dry cereal. You only need to add water when you want to mix it up.
- Keep an extra baby spoon and bib in your diaper bag.
- Always pack more dry cereal in your bag than you believe you might need. Baby may be hungrier than you thought she would be, or you might get stuck someplace with a hungry baby. This way, you'll be prepared!

Mealtime for Baby

- Some parents are concerned about *when* baby should be fed.
- Does she need one large meal and one small meal? Should meals be of equal size?
- Is one time of day better to feed her than another?
- It really doesn't make any difference, nutritionally. Offer her solids when she seems the hungriest.
- Your baby is probably the hungriest in the morning and may be in a good mood, so offering her a new food then might work best for you.
- Another benefit of morning feeding is that if she has any problem with the food, tummy upset should wear off before she goes to bed that night.
- If you breastfeed baby, offer food nearer to the end of the day.
- At this time, your milk supply is probably at its lowest, and baby may be more keen to eat.
- Offer her solids *between* breast feedings. Solid foods may interfere with the absorption of some nutrients in breast milk.
- If you bottlefeed, it may be a good idea to give her the larger feeding of cereal in the middle of the day to help her get through the day.
- You don't have to feed her solids at dinnertime if you give her solids in the morning and at lunch.

- At night, she can join you in her high chair. Give her a cracker to play with (she probably won't eat it) while you eat.
- When baby begins eating a more varied diet, you may decide to feed her the main meal at night.
- In this early exposure to solids, allow lots of time to feed baby.
- She'll want to play with her food, smear it, drop it and examine it closely.
- It's all part of the learning process!

Baby High Chairs

- Once baby is eating solids, it's time to think about a high chair.
- It may be one of the most used baby products you'll buy. You can feed baby in the high chair.
- She can sit in her high chair while the family eats.
- You may use it as an activity center when you're busy preparing a meal.
- When she's in her high chair, you know she's off the floor and out of harm's way.
- Many high chairs are adaptable to baby's age and developmental abilities.
- Some can even be made into a youth chair.
- Other types attach to the table; they save space and they're portable and less expensive than a regular high chair.

Choosing a High Chair to Suit Your Tastes

There is a wide variety of high chairs available on the market, so you should be able to find what you want. Whichever one you choose, it may be used by baby for 2 to 3 years. If you have other children, they may use it, too. So choose something sturdy that you can live with for a long time.

- You can choose from high chairs made of wood, plastic or metal.
- Some styles serve only one purpose—holding baby so she can eat. Others have a variety of uses.
- A wood high chair may be appealing, but it has some drawbacks.
  - ~ The seat may be too deep and the footrest too low for a small baby.
  - ~ If the tray is wood, it may be harder to clean and keep clean than plastic or metal.
  - ~ A wood chair may not fold up, so storing it and transporting it can be difficult.
- If you're looking for a simple high chair to serve baby's feeding needs, a basic metal-framed or plastic-framed model is fairly inexpensive.
- Metal or plastic-framed chairs are usually lightweight and collapsible. They're portable, too.
- Full-featured high chairs are often convenient to use and very comfortable for baby.
- Seats are well padded.

- Trays are easy to detach, and the entire chair cleans up easily.
- Some have reclining seat backs.
- Some adjust to baby's growth.
- Many have wheels for ease in moving.

Features to Consider in a High Chair

Below is a list of features you may want to think about before you buy a high chair.
- A wide base keeps it from tipping over easily.
- Seat is well padded and covered with sturdy plastic.
- There are no sharp edges.
- It's easy to clean.
- The tray is easy to attach and to remove—with one hand, if possible.
- The restraint system securely fastens baby across hips and between legs. Straps should be adjustable.
- If it has wheels, they lock to keep the chair from rolling while baby's in it.
- It adjusts so baby will be able to use it for a long time.
- It folds up compactly so it can be stored between uses or easily transported when eating away from home.
- Prices can range from $50 to $60 for a basic high chair into hundreds of dollars for a top-of-the-line, full-featured model.

Use a Drop Cloth

- Whether baby is eating a meal or just a snack, a drop cloth under her high chair may be a good investment.
- Putting a large, heavy-duty piece of plastic under her keeps your floor neat and makes cleanup easier.

- As baby is learning to eat, she is also experimenting with her food.
- She's sloppy, and a lot of what she "eats" actually ends up on the floor, so be prepared!

Changes in Baby's Bowels

- You may notice a change in baby's bowels now that she's eating more "grown-up" food.
- As you change the foods she eats, there will be a change in the consistency, color and frequency of her bowels. This is normal.
- It's not a sign of food allergies or food intolerance.
- In addition, until her first molars come in, she can't chew very well.
- As a result, some of the foods you feed her now may turn up in her stool looking much like they did when she ate them.
- When this occurs, don't be alarmed. There's nothing wrong with her digestion.
- Until her digestive system matures, you'll discover her stools may reflect the various foods she eats.
- As she gets older and begins eating different foods, when you feed her carrots, spinach or beets, you may see yellow, green or red stools.
- If she eats oat-circle cereal pieces, her stools may be a sandy color.
- Cucumber and tomato seeds and unchewed raisins may show up in her bowel movements.

FROM A MOM'S PERSPECTIVE

To me, breastfeeding was the most intelligent choice for my children. I dislike the chemicals in processed foods, and I believe there are too many chemicals in the foods we eat. When I breastfed my babies, I watched everything I put in my mouth so I wouldn't pass along bad things to them. I think that breastfed babies receive the ultimate nutrition from their moms! *Jane*

- One way to help deal with the situation is to make sure foods you give her are easy to digest.
- Chop, mash, purée, dice and blend foods that she may have difficulty with.
- These foods will also be safer for her to eat.

Is Baby Enthusiastic About Solids?

- Many babies take to solids and eat solid food with gusto from the time they are first introduced to cereal. Other babies don't like the taste or texture of solid food and refuse to eat it.
- If your baby decides she doesn't want to eat, don't fight with her about it.
- It may be a good idea to make the decision now that you will *never* fight with your child about food—at any age!
- When baby refuses to eat, continue offering her a spoonful of cereal at each meal.

- Your purpose in offering her solids is to introduce her to the taste and texture of food.
- If she won't eat, call your pediatrician for advice.
- He or she may suggest you wait a couple of weeks, then try again.

Baby's Eating Habits around 6 Months of Age

Taking in Less Formula or Breast Milk

- As baby begins to take in more nutrition from solid foods, she may begin to cut back somewhat on her intake of formula or breast milk. This is normal.
- If she is breastfed, she may do this on her own.
- If she is bottlefed, she may need some help.
- Ask your pediatrician for advice on how much formula or breast milk baby should be drinking.
- Although you want her to eat solid foods, you don't want her to give up her other important nutrition sources.
- Neither do you want her to take in too many calories.
- It's best to work this out with help from baby's doctor.

Is Baby Getting Enough Nourishment?

- By around 6 months of age, babies need about 800 calories a day—from a combination of formula or breast milk *and* solid foods.
- If she's taking in formula or breast milk and eats the various solid foods she can manage, she'll get enough

calories. You probably don't have to worry that she isn't getting enough nourishment.

- The best indications she is eating enough are her growth and well-being.
- If she's growing and putting on weight, and she is energetic, she's getting enough nourishment.
- Remember, feeding her solids at this time isn't for the nutrition she receives. It's more for socialization, learning how to eat and introducing her to the taste and texture of eating "grown-up" food.

Food Is not Just for Eating

- Eating is becoming more enjoyable for baby because she can manipulate a few food items.
- She likes to feed herself a cracker or small piece of bread.
- She wants to taste food, but she also wants to play with it, squeeze it, smell it, crumble it, mash it and smear it.
- Being messy is part of her learning process.

Is Baby Ready for a Cup?

- Around 6 months of age, your baby may show interest in drinking from a cup.
- Help her hold a cup, and see how she responds.

- If she seems interested and willing to drink from it, use it as a *supplement* to bottlefeeding or breastfeeding. Don't use it as a replacement.
- Spillproof cups, made especially for a baby, are available in many stores.
- They usually have two handles for baby to grip and a cover with a spout.
- It's even better if the cup has a weighted bottom. Using one of these cups helps keep baby from spilling liquid all over herself.
- You'll be glad she can drink from a cup, too, when she's thirsty and a cup is the only thing available!
- Below are some other helpful tips to get her started.
  - ~ When she takes her first sip, she should be sitting in her high chair or infant seat. Show her how to drink from one of her cups. Then help her drink from hers. After she gets the hang of it, let her experiment.
  - ~ Put a few sips of water in the cup while she's learning. It's not as messy or as wasteful as using juice, breast milk or formula.
  - ~ A small amount is also easier for her to handle.
  - ~ It may not take long for baby to become adept at drinking from a cup. She'll master it quickly if she has your help.
  - ~ Don't get frustrated if it takes her awhile to catch on.
  - ~ For some babies, it's months before they master drinking from a cup.

~ If she doesn't seem interested or ready, wait for a time, then try again.
~ Some babies are not ready to drink from a cup until they're 8 or 9 months old.
~ Drinking from a cup is an important transition for baby.
~ Smile and praise her when she's practicing.

Her Taste Buds Are Developing

• Your baby has hundreds more taste buds for sweets than you do.
• That's one reason she loves sweet-tasting foods, such as applesauce or mashed bananas.
• Don't offer her foods sweetened with sugar or any other sweetener. She doesn't need them.
• The fruits and vegetables she eats that taste sweet naturally will satisfy her for a long time.

What Baby Is Eating

• Your baby is eating larger amounts of cereal now.
• Until this time, you've given her only formula or breast milk and cereal.
• Baby now takes three to five servings of formula or breast milk a day; each serving is probably 6 to 8 ounces.
• She's also eating two feedings of cereal a day; each feeding is probably about 2 to 4 tablespoons.

- Because her appetite is increasing, it may be time to add a little more variety to her diet.
- If your baby has tried all the different varieties of baby cereal and seems ready for more food, you may be able to add a few new foods.
- Call your pediatrician *before* you feed baby more than just cereal. He or she may have particular suggestions or advice for your baby.
- It's best to begin with strained fruit and vegetables.
- You can also offer your baby fruit juice in a cup.
- Finger foods, such as toast and plain crackers, are also good to try.
- Suggested foods to offer baby at this time, and the amounts of each, are listed below:
  - ~ bread or toast, unbuttered—1/2 slice
  - ~ crackers—2
  - ~ fruit—2 to 3 tablespoons, 2 servings a day
  - ~ fruit juice (diluted with equal amount of water)—3 ounces, 1 serving a day from a cup
  - ~ vegetables—2 to 3 tablespoons, 2 servings a day

Foods to Avoid with Baby

Some foods should not be given to a baby under the age of 1 year. Below is a list of various foods to avoid and an explanation of why each could be harmful to your baby.

- Any food that is a choking hazard; see the box on page 94.

- Cow's milk because the proteins are too hard for baby to digest.
- Spinach, beets, carrots and turnips prepared at home. Each contains large amounts of nitrates and could cause anemia. Prepared baby food is OK because manufacturers remove harmful substances.
- Egg whites because the protein is too hard to digest. They may also cause allergic reactions. It's OK to feed baby egg yolks.

Choking Hazards to Avoid

When baby begins eating finger foods, some foods should be completely avoided, no matter how small they are cut, because they are common choking hazards. Do *not* feed your baby any of the following until she's quite a bit older (at least 1 year of age or older for some other foods):

- cut-up hot dogs
- peanut butter
- grapes
- popcorn
- nuts
- chewing gum
- hard candy
- ice cubes
- marshmallows
- potato chips
- tortilla chips
- raisins
- raw carrots

Adding Fruits and Vegetables to Baby's Diet

After eating baby cereal, it can take some time for baby to get used to eating fruits and vegetables. Even strained baby food can have a strong taste after such bland fare.

- When making your choices at the store, buy strained fruits and vegetables.
- They are a little easier for baby to swallow and to digest.
- She doesn't have to chew any of the strained variety.
- Offer baby only one new strained fruit or vegetable *each week*.
- You can see if she has any problems with the food, such as an allergic reaction to it or trouble digesting it.
- Give her 1 to 2 tablespoons of either a fruit or vegetable at two meals when you first offer it. You want to work up to 2 to 3 tablespoons at each meal.
- If baby doesn't like the food you offer her, wait a couple of days before trying it again.
- Let her continue to eat what she was eating before you introduced the new food.
- When selecting juice for baby, buy vitamin C-fortified apple, pear or grape juice.
- Avoid orange juice or grapefruit juice at this time. They're too acidic for her.
- Dilute all juices you give baby. Add as much water to the juice as the amount of juice. If you want to give baby 4 ounces of fluid, mix 2 ounces of juice with 2 ounces of water.
- Offer her the juice in a cup.

Are Fruits Better than Vegetables?

- Vegetables are more nutritious than fruits. However, offering vegetables before you offer fruits may not entice your baby to eat them.
- Fruits taste better, so baby may accept them more readily in the beginning.
- At this point in baby's life, you aren't trying to meet all of her nutritional needs with solids. That's the main reason you continue giving her formula or breast milk.
- The goal at this time is to teach baby to swallow foods with different textures.
- You will probably have more success feeding her fruits than vegetables.
- When you introduce vegetables, try the sweeter ones first. Carrots and sweet potatoes are good choices. She may not like them as well as the fruit, but keep trying.
- If you keep offering them to her, she'll learn to like vegetables.

Some Fruits and Vegetables Baby Might Like

- Most of the foods you offer baby are normal ones you probably think of when you think about baby foods, such as applesauce and pears. Both are great for baby. Applesauce has a great texture, and it's low in citric acid. Pears are easily digested and a good source of potassium.

- Some foods you may *not* think about giving baby are ones you may eat yourself. Next time you have them, try them with baby.
  - ~ Sweet potatoes and winter squash are often favorites with baby because of their taste, texture and color.
  - ~ They both contain beta-carotene.
  - ~ Thoroughly mash the cooked food.
  - ~ Don't add butter, sugar, salt or anything else to it. It's better for her to try a food without anything extra added.
  - ~ A ripe avocado is great. You can feed her a little right out of the shell!
  - ~ Avocados contain lots of vitamins and minerals— A, B_6, E, folic acid, niacin, magnesium, potassium and phosphorous.
  - ~ The texture of an avocado is unique, and the flavor is mild.
- Never give baby a large amount of any new food. Let her have a few tastes, then wait to see if she has any reactions.
- As baby eats more fruits and vegetables, offer her vegetables before fruit in each meal.
- It's better for baby to be a little hungry when you feed her vegetables.
- A baby likes the tastes of sweets, so even if she's eaten some food, she doesn't have to be as hungry to eat her fruit.

Getting Baby to Eat

- Offer new foods fairly often, and urge baby to try them, but don't get into a battle with her if she doesn't eat them.
- She doesn't need to eat everything she's given.
- She can get filled up quite quickly because she has a tiny stomach.
- Try to make meal times enjoyable for her and for you.
- When she loses interest or gets fussy, she's finished.

When Baby Refuses Food

- Don't be surprised or frustrated when baby spits out a new food you offer her.
- All babies do this at one time or another.
- It's the newness of the food that causes baby to spit it out. It doesn't taste bad or smell bad.
- If baby repeats her actions more than a few times, wait for a while before offering the food again.
- It may take awhile for her to get used to it.

Some Tips for Feeding Baby

- When you feed jarred baby food, don't feed baby out of the jar.
- Take out only enough for one feeding.
- Put the rest back in the refrigerator to prevent bacterial growth.

- Buy small jars of baby food when you're traveling. If you can't refrigerate leftovers, throw them away.
- Or buy dried baby food and mix only the amount needed for one meal.
- To help baby learn to drink from a cup, give her juice in a cup.
- She probably enjoys the taste of the juice and may be more willing to drink juice, rather than formula or breast milk, from a cup.
- Buy the spillproof kind of infant cup that holds 6 to 10 ounces.
- Some have handles for baby to grasp.
- With most cups, the top doesn't come off easily, so when baby drops it, it stays sealed.
- Choose a cup that has a self-sealing valve. Juice stays in the cup, even when its turned upside down!
- Use a rubber- or plastic-coated baby spoon. Now that she is closer to teething, a baby spoon with a rubber or heavy plastic coating over the bowl area may be easier and more comfortable for her to use.

Your Baby's Food Experience at 8 to 9 Months Old

Baby Wants to Feed Herself

- As baby gets older, you may find she wants to try feeding herself.
- She wants to eat foods she can easily hold in her hand.

- She may thwart your efforts to feed her because she wants to do it herself.
- Unfortunately, she doesn't have the coordination.
- Baby can't guide the spoon to her mouth on a consistent basis, so it's too soon to let her try to feed herself with a utensil.
- Keep giving her finger foods to help her develop the skills she needs so she can feed herself in the not-too-distant future.

Baby's Pincer Grasp Is Developing

- Baby is developing her pincer grasp, which allows her to pick up food with her thumb and forefinger.
- Feeding herself becomes enjoyable.
- She can't use utensils yet—she's not coordinated enough.
- Eating food with her fingers is easier and a lot more fun.

Finger Foods

- If you haven't started feeding baby finger foods, about 8 to 9 months is a good time to begin.
- The object of giving baby finger foods is to help her learn to feed herself.
- Because she can't use a spoon effectively, finger foods allow her to practice.
- *Finger foods* are small, baby bite-sized pieces of food.

- Crackers, teething crackers, pieces of toast, pieces of cheese, small bits of meat, pieces of soft tortilla and well-cooked pieces of pasta or macaroni are good finger foods to begin with. Also see the discussion below.
- Offer her many different kinds of food.
- Let her touch, taste and smell them.
- Remember to be patient. It takes her much longer to eat when she feeds herself.

Grain-Based Finger Foods Are Good Choices

- If baby wants to feed herself, offer her some grain-based foods.
- These foods become mushy in her mouth, which makes chewing and swallowing them easier for her.
- Baby crackers, well-cooked pasta (not al dente), bread and oat-circle cereal pieces are good choices. These foods are easier to chew and to swallow.
- They also offer many of the same nutrients—B vitamins and iron—that are found in infant cereals.
- When you serve baby these foods and she eats them, it helps you out, too.

- You'll be able to eliminate one or two servings of cereal each day from her meal plan.

Giving Baby Sweets

- You may wonder about giving baby sweets.
- Will offering them cause her to develop a sweet tooth?
- Will it affect the foods she chooses or wants to eat?
- Are sweets empty calories?
- If you give your baby sweets, you give her calories that have little nutritional value.
- However, it's not a problem if you don't do this too often and don't give her large amounts.
- A small taste is all she really needs.
- If you deny her *all* sweets, you could be setting the stage for eating problems in the future.
- As she gets older, it may be hard to avoid giving her *any* sweets.
- If you don't give them to her, someone else might, such as grandma or a sibling.

Don't Give Baby Honey!

Caution: Do *not* give your baby honey or foods made with honey during her first 2 years! Although honey is a natural substance, there could be a risk of baby getting botulism from eating it. See the discussion of botulism on page 141. Baby's digestive system is not ready to handle the botulism spores sometimes found in honey.

- There will be times that a little sweet food is acceptable, so you might want to allow her a treat.
- During her 1st year, don't give her ice cream as a sweet treat.
- The milk protein is too hard for her to digest.
- Control what sweets she receives, how much she gets and how often she eats them.

Suggestions for Offering New Foods to Your Older Baby

- As your baby gets older, she needs a more balanced diet.
- She has nearly depleted the iron supplies she received before birth.
- She must now get the mineral from other sources. If baby drinks iron-fortified formula, she's getting the iron she needs.
- If she's breastfeeding, she may need extra iron.

- Check with your pediatrician before you make any changes, such as giving her vitamins with iron.
- As you begin to expand her diet, she may not take to a new food immediately.
- When that happens, combine a small portion of the new food with one she's been eating.
- For example, introduce green beans to baby with her sweet potatoes.
- If she normally eats 3 teaspoons of sweet potatoes, put 2 teaspoons of sweet potatoes in a bowl and add 1 teaspoon of green beans.
- The next day, add a little more of the green beans to a little less of the sweet potatoes.
- Keep doing this until she's eating only the green beans.
- This practice allows baby to get used to a new taste gradually.
- It may also make it easier for you to spot any allergic reactions.

Forbidden Foods for an Older Baby

As baby becomes better at eating, you'll be considering different foods to add to her diet. Once she can eat more than puréed food, you may mistakenly believe she can eat anything. She can't.

- Be cautious with the foods listed on page 105 until your baby has a full set of teeth and you feel certain she won't choke on food.
- See the list of choking hazards on page 94.

- Below is a list of different foods that might be too difficult for baby to eat.
- It may be a good idea *not* to offer baby any of these foods until she is much older (probably over 1 year old).
  - ~ Raw foods that snap into small, hard pieces. These include celery, carrots, green peppers, hard apples, hard pears, jicama.
  - ~ Hot dogs, sausages or bratwurst. Slicing this type of meat doesn't make it safer. If you want to offer your baby these foods, remove all the skin from the meat. Cut each piece into lengthwise quarters, then slice each quarter into 1/4 inch segments.
  - ~ Chunks of meat.
  - ~ Peanut butter of any sort. See the discussion on page 113.
  - ~ Fruit with seeds or pits. Core then remove pits or seeds. Mash the fruit before feeding baby.
  - ~ Fruit that has thick skin, such as plums. Skin, remove pits or seeds, then mash fruit before feeding baby.
  - ~ Seeds, even small ones, such as sunflower seeds.
  - ~ Olives, cherries or grapes.
  - ~ Any food that is smooth and round that she could easily choke on.
  - ~ Anything that might have bones in it, such as fish.
- *A word of advice:* Teach your baby to say "aaah." If you find baby has something in her mouth that you want to see and/or remove, you can do it quickly when she says "aaah."

Baby May Play with Her Food

- Your baby may spend more time playing with and smearing her food than she does eating it.
- You may want her to stop and to attend to the task of eating.
- However, as messy as she may be at this time, let her continue.
- Playing with her food helps baby become aware of the various textures of different foods.
- It's her way of exploring and learning.
- Let her experiment with her food.
- You don't have to let her become destructive, but a little testing won't do any harm.
- She'll find her mouth when she gets hungry.

Feeding Tips as She Gets Older

By the time baby is about 8 months old, she may be eating solids fairly well. She's becoming more adept at eating different foods. Below are some tips to keep in mind when feeding baby.

- If baby has any food left in her bowl, throw it out when she's finished.
- Don't add any sweeteners to baby's food, especially honey!
- When you warm her food, check it before you serve it to her. Stir and taste before serving.

- Don't put fruit juice in a bottle; it may stay in contact with her teeth for a longer time, which could cause cavities.
- Even if you've already fed her, make baby a part of the family at mealtimes. It's good for her to be exposed to the interactions of family members during this time.

If You Have Problems Feeding Baby

When baby is about 9 months old, she may begin refusing to eat because she wants to feed herself.

- If baby decides she doesn't want you to feed her or she wants to eat what she can put in her mouth, consider some of the following foods.
- They allow her to feed herself, and they're not too messy.
- Foods that are easy for her to eat and to feed herself include:
  ~ small bits of meat, such as ground meat (cook thoroughly!)
  ~ small pieces of macaroni or spaghetti
  ~ baby bite-size chunks of soft foods, such as mashed yams or mashed bananas
- Be sure the foods you feed your baby do not cause her to choke.
- She may not realize how much she can put in her mouth. It's easy for her to put too much into her mouth and choke or gag herself, so keep an eye on her!

Don't Get Uptight

Don't get too uptight at mealtime. If you do, researchers believe it could lead to feeding problems for baby.

- A baby often gets rambunctious when she's eating.
- Stay cool, calm and collected when she does.
- Within reason, follow baby's wishes.
- If she wants to help out with the spoon, let her give it a try.
- If she wants to eat with her fingers, it's probably OK.

Trends in Baby Foods

- Some baby-food manufacturers have made the decision to offer foods that are grown without synthetic pesticides or fertilizers.
- Their baby-food products are organically produced.
- Baby-food producers are doing this because consumers are interested in feeding baby naturally grown foods.
- If this is important to you, read the labels on the baby foods you choose, and talk to your grocer.

Are You Interested in Making Your Own Baby Food?

Many parents want to make their own baby food. You can do it and maintain baby's health by keeping a few things in mind. Follow the suggestions listed below.

- Thoroughly cook the foods you choose.
- Purée the cooked foods so they are very mushy.

- Use only fresh foods.
- Don't add salt, sugar, spices or anything extra to the food.
- Good choices to start with include sweet potatoes, peas and squash.
- Make only a little at a time, so you don't have to store it.
- If you make more than you need, store leftovers in a sealed container in the refrigerator.
- Keep leftovers no longer than 2 days.

Puréeing Protein Foods

- If you want to purée some tender beef or chicken for baby, go ahead.
- Thoroughly cook the meat with broth or water, then purée.
- Mash the yolk of a boiled egg.
- Serve any of these foods once a day.
- You can move on to finely minced protein when baby eats mashed food without any problems.
- Don't worry about whether she's getting enough nutrition. Baby's protein needs are still quite low.

- Her nutritional needs are still being met with formula or breast milk.

Baby's Eating Lots of Different Foods

By this time, your baby may be eating lots of different foods. She is still taking in 24 to 32 ounces of formula or breast milk each day.
- However, she's probably started tasting (and eating) some other new foods.
- By this point, her daily nutritional plan may consist of:
  - ~ 1/2 cup each of cheese, plain yogurt or plain cottage cheese
  - ~ 2 or 3 servings of 2 to 4 tablespoons of iron-fortified baby cereal
  - ~ 2 or 3 servings of 1/2 slice of bread or 2 crackers
  - ~ 2 servings of 3 to 4 tablespoons of fruit
  - ~ 3 ounces of fruit juice from a cup—dilute it with water before serving
  - ~ 2 or 3 servings of 3 to 4 tablespoons of vegetables
  - ~ 2 servings of 3 to 4 tablespoons of protein, including chicken, beef, pork, cooked dry beans or egg yolks
- If you offer baby any meat products, they should be strained or finely minced.
- Feed her only *one* new meat a week. When you offer eggs, just give her the yolks.
- Some babies are sensitive to egg whites until after they are 1 year old.

Your Pet's Food

A word of caution: If you have animals and keep their food on the floor, keep an eye on baby when she's near it. Eating a piece or two of dog food or cat food isn't a problem, but you don't want her to eat it on a regular basis. This advisory also applies to the pet's water dish. Children have been known to drown in 1 inch of water, so a pet's water dish could be dangerous. Use caution with your curious baby.

When Baby Eats Food Off the Floor

- As your baby begins to eat different foods, you will be faced with many challenges.
- One is eating food off the floor.
- As diligent as you may be about cleaning up after her, you may miss something. It's normal.
- When baby crawls around on the floor, she's sure to find something you missed.
- You may be concerned that the oat-circle cereal pieces or the macaroni you missed may harm baby when she eats it.
- Most experts agree that if baby occasionally eats food off the floor, it probably won't harm her.
- The exception is a household with pets that are not house-trained.
- Food off a floor contaminated with pet urine or feces could cause problems for baby.

- In general, however, the germs on your floors aren't the ones that make baby sick, so don't get panicky when your baby eats food she finds on the floor.

Breastfeeding Babies May Forgo Middle-of-the-Night Feedings

- Around 9 months of age, a healthy breastfeeding infant can probably skip her middle-of-the-night feed.
- She should be able to go from late at night to early morning without too much trouble.
- However, she may resist your efforts to skip the middle-of-the-night feeding.
- To help deal with the situation, let dad go in when she wakes up.
- Baby may fuss for a few nights, but she'll soon settle down.
- If you have any problems, contact your pediatrician for advice.

Offering Her a Cup

- If baby has been bottlefeeding, she may show less interest in it now.
- Offer her some formula (not cow's milk!) in a cup.
- Many babies are ready to be weaned at about 9 months of age.
- Don't be surprised, however, if she changes her mind next month.

- Her willingness will probably reappear by the time she's a year old.

Peanut Allergies on the Rise

Peanut allergies seem to be on the rise. This allergy accounts for many food-induced deaths.

- The number of children allergic to peanuts *doubled* in the years between 1980 and 1994; however, only 1% of Americans have this allergy.
- Some experts believe the increase has occurred because more children are being exposed to peanut protein before age 3.
- A child's immature immune system may consider the protein harmful and develop antibodies to it. This triggers an allergic reaction.
- Researchers advise parents to delay introducing peanut butter to children if there is any family history of peanut allergies.
- *Caution:* To help avoid developing the allergy in *any* child, do not offer your child peanut butter or other products made with peanuts until she's 3, and do not eat peanuts if you breastfeed.
- It isn't just peanuts and peanut butter that can cause problems; foods made without peanut products can also be contaminated.
- If food is mixed or stirred with utensils that were used with peanut-protein foods, they can be cross-contaminated if utensils are not thoroughly cleaned.

FROM A MOM'S PERSPECTIVE

I breastfed all four of my children. When my first baby was born, money was pretty tight for us. Breastfeeding was the most economical way for me to go! We didn't have to buy formula for the first year, which saved us a lot of money (from what my friends told me). I liked it so much, I breastfed my other three kids for a year each, too. *Polly*

- If you know your child has a peanut allergy, ask when you eat out if food might have come in contact with peanuts or peanut products.
- Symptoms of an allergic reaction to peanuts include hives, diarrhea, a stomach ache, swelling in the throat, wheezing, vomiting and faintness or unconsciousness. Hives or swelling may also appear when a nut comes in contact with the skin.
- It's important to read labels. Many foods contain peanuts, peanut oil or other peanut products, so check labels very closely. Peanuts may be near the end of the list.
- Unexpected sources of peanut protein include the following foods:
  ~ bakery items
  ~ potato chips
  ~ packaged cheese and crackers
  ~ many chocolate candies—not only the peanut varieties

- ~ chili sauces at restaurants
- ~ gravies at restaurants
- ~ Asian, Thai, Chinese and African dishes often use peanut butter and other peanut proteins
- Discuss the situation with your pediatrician if you or your partner have a family history of peanut allergy or if you are concerned.

Good Food Choices for Your Baby at 9 to 10 Months

- Some good choices to offer a baby who is 9 to 10 months old include bananas and ripe apricots.
- Well-cooked vegetables, such as carrots, yams, potatoes and peas are also tasty.
- If you want to offer meat, choose soft meats, such as turkey and well-cooked stew beef.
- Cut food into small enough pieces so baby can gum them. Cut them about the size of her thumbnail.
- Food pieces should be small enough that if baby swallows a piece whole, she won't choke.
- Your baby may be even less interested in drinking her formula or breastfeeding now.
- Offering her 1 or 2 tablespoons of a protein food every day helps her get the nutrition she needs.
- Meat, cheese, egg yolk or tofu (microwaved for 15 seconds, then cooled) are other interesting choices.

- Offer her foods of various textures. Slippery spaghetti, sticky mashed potatoes, crunchy oat-circle cereal pieces—each one offers something different.

Citrus Juice

By 9 to 10 months of age, if your baby hasn't had any problems with the foods you've offered her, you might want to try a citrus juice.

- Limit the *total* amount of *all juice* you give her to 4 ounces a day.
- Be sure you cut the juice with at least as much water— 2 ounces of juice to 2 ounces of water.
- Give her the juice in a cup.
- You can offer her orange juice, but don't give her grapefruit juice yet. It may be too hard on her tummy.
- Another good selection is a small amount of citrus juice mixed with another juice, such as apple juice or pear juice.

Begin Adding Lumpier Foods

By the time baby is 10 months old, she may be ready to start eating lumpier puréed foods. Some new table foods may also be offered.

- You're probably already giving her crackers and bits of cheese.
- Add cooked rice and baked potato removed from its skin. Be sure pieces are no larger than a green pea.

- Offer baby a spoon, and let her feed herself.
- Don't give her the baby spoons you've been using to feed her. Choose a spoon with a fairly large handle so she can grasp it easily.
- Don't be concerned about the mess she creates.
- It'll take lot of practice before she can get the spoon and its contents to her mouth.

When Baby Gags on Foods

Some parents hesitate to add lumpier foods to baby's diet because they don't want her to gag or choke. However, doing this could interfere with baby's learning to eat properly.

- One of the goals of feeding solids to a baby during the first year is to teach tongue control.
- Your baby needs to learn how to push food around in her mouth with her tongue.
- To do this, she needs to progress through the different textures of food—from strained to puréed to lumpy to small bits of "real food," such as well-cooked meats and vegetables.
- If she doesn't progress through these foods, she may have problems later.
- You may not know exactly when to offer the next level of food.
- Experts suggest offering her foods of the next level in manageable bites when she masters a level. For example, when she's eating puréed food without problems, begin introducing lumpier foods.

- Don't be alarmed when baby gags on a food every once in awhile.
- When she's learning to swallow, she gags as a normal way to protect herself.
- Some babies have a more sensitive gag reflex than others and may gag more easily.
- If baby gags consistently, contact your pediatrician. It may indicate a problem.

Feeding Baby from 10 Months to 1 Year

Can Yogurt Help Prevent Diarrhea?

One study followed babies between 10 and 18 months old. In the study, some babies were fed yogurt, while others were not.

- Each baby's stool was evaluated throughout the study.
- Researchers found that babies who ate yogurt had more "good" bacteria in their intestinal tracts.
- Good bacteria in the intestine is a plus for baby. Too much "bad" bacteria can cause diarrhea.
- Findings suggest that if a baby has some yogurt in her diet on a regular basis, it may help keep harmful bacteria from growing, thus helping to prevent diarrhea.
- A bonus to eating yogurt is its calcium content. It also contains riboflavin, potassium and magnesium. Baby needs all these minerals in her diet.
- Yogurt is also a good transitional food for your baby.

FROM A MOM'S PERSPECTIVE

I don't think I would have breastfed my first child (and the other one, too), if I hadn't received so much help in the hospital. My baby had trouble latching on, and it hurt when he sucked. I asked one really nice nurse to help me, and she spent hours with me. We talked about different things to do, such as ways to hold my baby, and she arranged for me to watch some videos that covered all sorts of things about breastfeeding. I learned a lot in a short time, and being successful in the hospital helped me be more confident when I got home. *Carly*

- You don't have to feed her large amounts of yogurt. A few teaspoons of *plain* (not flavored or sweetened) yogurt might be beneficial for her.
- Try it—you may be surprised how much she likes it.

Don't Let Baby Have Fruit with Seeds

As baby gets teeth, she may soon be eating larger pieces of apples, watermelon and grapes.

- It's a good idea to be very careful with these fruits because they have seeds.
- An inhaled seed from fruit can be very dangerous.
- Under age 5, a child can easily suck a seed into her airway.
- An inhaled seed can block breathing and cause choking.

- And if a seed remains in the lung, it may cause an infection.
- The best plan is to get rid of all seeds before giving a piece of fruit to baby.
- Don't give her sunflower or pumpkin seeds until she's at least 5 years old.
- If your child begins to cough or to wheeze after eating some fruit, she may have inhaled a seed.
- Call your pediatrician; he or she may want a chest X-ray taken.
- If a seed is found, it may need to be removed by a specialist with a tool called a *bronchoscope.*

Keep Feeding Her Breast Milk or Formula

- You are now probably offering your baby more solid food at mealtime.
- However, even at 10 months, when she's eating at least two meals a day, breast milk or formula should still be supplying much of her nutrition.
- Offer breast milk or a bottle between meals, when she's hungry.

Mealtime Fun

Is mealtime with baby a hassle? Is it messy? It may help if you try to make mealtime fun for your growing baby. Make feeding easier on you and baby by trying some of the suggestions on the opposite page.

- Feed yourself first. Eat in an exaggerated way. Show how much you like the food. She'll probably want to try it if she thinks *you* like it.

- "Open the door." When baby is hungry, but not *too* hungry, open your mouth wide. Say "open the door." Once she opens her mouth, put the food in.

- Up and in. When feeding baby, put a spoonful of the food in her mouth as you lift the spoon up. Her upper lip will clean the spoon, which helps food stay in her mouth!

- Don't push it. If baby doesn't want to eat a meal, she'll be OK. Sometimes she just doesn't feel like eating. She may be teething, and her mouth is a little sore. She may be getting a cold. Or maybe she doesn't like what you're offering. Skip solids for a meal or two, then offer them again.

- Occupy her hands. Some babies want to reach for and take the spoon themselves. Some like to pour their liquids on the high-chair tray. Some want to drop food on the floor. Give baby a spoon of her own when you feed her. Use plates and bowls that attach to the tray. Some high chairs have activity bars that will entertain her. Use whatever methods work best for you.

Thirst Quenchers

As baby is getting older, your pediatrician may recommend giving her more fluids.

- There are many liquids you can offer her. Some are better than others.

- Below is a comparison of various liquids you might be thinking about offering baby.
  - ~ water—one of the best because it doesn't contain sugar, caffeine or flavorings
  - ~ fruit pieces—contain a lot of water, often as high as 85%
  - ~ juice—often contains lots of sugar
  - ~ soda—usually high in sugar and caffeine
  - ~ ice pops—often contain flavorings and sugar
  - ~ sports drinks—contain sugar and electrolytes, which are usually unnecessary

Can Baby Eat a Vegetarian Diet?

Some parents choose to feed their families a vegetarian diet, whether for religious or personal reasons. Many want to know if a baby can get the nutrients she needs from a vegetarian meal plan.

- A baby can be fed a vegetarian diet if she is offered a wide variety of foods.
- Different vegetarian eating plans require special considerations.
- If you choose to feed your baby a vegetarian diet, be sure you discuss it first with your pediatrician.
- It can be difficult for baby to get all the nutrients she needs.
- You may need assistance from a dietician in meeting her nutritional requirements.

- Your pediatrician will also advise you about any special concerns or needs.
- The *ovo-lacto diet* includes dairy products and eggs.
- When baby is eating solid foods, be sure she receives adequate amounts of food that contain protein, iron and B_{12}.
- However, don't feed her any egg whites until she is at least a year old; this helps her avoid developing an allergy to eggs.
- Dairy foods are part of the *lacto-vegetarian diet,* but eggs are not.
- Adequate amounts of food that contain protein, iron and B_{12} are necessary in this diet plan.
- The *vegan diet* does not include any animal products, such as dairy foods or eggs.
- When solids are introduced to baby, any vegetarian diet must contain adequate amounts of calcium, protein, iron and B_{12}.
- You can meet these needs by giving baby iron-enriched grains and cereals. Serving them with foods that contain vitamin C helps with iron absorption.
- Soy products are rich in protein, and many are enriched with calcium and B_{12}.
- Soy products baby may like include tofu, soy cheese and soy milk.
- By around 7 months, you can start adding puréed beans, lentils and split peas as other sources of protein to baby's diet.

Foods Baby Is Eating Now

By the time your baby reaches 11 months old, she is eating lots of different things.

- She probably eats infant cereal or other grain foods at all three meals. Portions for each meal are 1/4 cup cereal, 1/4 slice of bread or 1/4 cup of cooked pasta.
- Baby is eating soft fruits at two meals a day and soft veggies at two meals a day. Portions of each at a meal are 2 to 3 tablespoons.
- Baby isn't eating that much meat, though—about 1 to 2 tablespoons at two meals a day.
- One way to provide her with the nutrition she needs in foods she likes is to make combination dishes.
- Some good choices include macaroni and cheese, a casserole of meat, rice and a vegetable or jarred combination baby foods.
- Remember when you cook to leave out the spices. At this age, baby may not like them.

When Baby Is a Picky Eater

- From a very early age, some babies are picky eaters.
- When a baby is a picky eater, she refuses certain foods, eats only a couple of foods or won't eat at all.
- Some foods you offer her supply a lot of nutrition.
- Even if she doesn't get all of her nutrition in one sitting, eating these foods helps her eat a balanced diet.

- Offer her yogurt, which is rich in calcium, protein and vitamin B_{12}.
- Egg yolks contain protein, riboflavin and vitamins A, B_{12} and K.
- Cereals are loaded with vitamins, zinc, iron, magnesium and folate.
- Beans and lentils are high-protein sources of iron and folate.
- Tomatoes are rich in vitamin C and lycopene.
- Below are some tips that might help you deal with a picky eater. Use what works best for you and your baby.
  - *Give baby enough time to eat.* Some babies need more time to eat. Try setting aside an extra 15 minutes for mealtime.
  - *Feed her first.* If she drinks a lot, she may not have room in her tummy for food. Offer food first, then breastfeed or give her a bottle later.
  - *Don't let her snack too much during the day.* If you give her snacks whenever she's hungry, she won't want to eat at mealtime. Schedule snacks for certain times and stick with the schedule.
  - *Keep introducing new foods.* Your baby may need time to adjust to a new food, a new taste or a new texture. Wait a few days after she refuses something, then try again. Sometimes you may have to try up to a dozen times before baby will eat a food.
  - *Give her the same foods if she'll eat them.* If baby wants to eat only macaroni and cheese for a while,

FROM A MOM'S PERSPECTIVE

My baby wasn't a good eater when I first started breastfeeding her. When I took her to her 2-week checkup, she hadn't gained much weight at all. My pediatrician suggested I talk with a lactation consultant. She explained that these people were available to help new mothers with the problems they might have when they started feeding their baby. She had a list of consultants that she gave me. Before I called anyone, I contacted my OB-GYN to see what he had to say about it. The nurse had me read the list I had and told me they were all good. I called one and made an appointment to visit with her. She gave me lots of information and advice and even let me borrow a couple of videos. It sure made a difference! *Rosemary*

 let her. She will eventually tire of it. It's OK to take this approach for a few weeks. It won't hurt her.

~ *Set a good example.* When you eat a healthy diet and a good selection of foods, so will your baby.

~ *If you don't like it, don't let her know.* We know that certain foods, broccoli for example, may taste great to some and awful to others. Or there may be some foods that you just can't stand. Keep your attitudes to yourself. Let baby try different foods and decide on her own whether she likes them.

~ *Her appetite may be small.* Some babies don't have large appetites. Don't expect her to eat a lot or to eat often. Let baby set some of the parameters of her eating. Pushing too much food on her when she can't eat may cause problems. Her stomach is only the size of her small fist, so it probably doesn't hold as much as you might expect.

~ *Don't make mealtimes a hassle.* These interactions can cause lots of problems, now and later. You may teach her that mealtime battles are a way of gaining your attention. Ignore the situation when you can. Within reason, let baby decide what to eat and how much she wants.

Trust Baby to Eat What She Needs

- Unless your baby is sick, trust her to eat what she needs.
- As long as you offer her a variety of nutritious foods, she'll get the vitamins, minerals and calories she needs to help her grow healthy and strong.
- The best measure of how she's doing is whether she's growing and thriving.
- If she's doing well, she's probably getting what she needs from the breast milk or formula you give her and from the food she eats.

Baby's Food Needs as the End of the 1st Year Draws Near

Your baby's nutritional needs change somewhat as she nears the end of her 1st year. In a few weeks, she may be drinking whole milk. Be sure to discuss this with her doctor. Your baby's nutritional plan may closely resemble the one listed below.

- Baby is eating yogurt, cheese and cottage cheese. Offer her a little plain vanilla ice cream as a special treat. She should have four servings of dairy foods a day. Serving size varies from $1/4$ cup to $1/2$ cup.
- Six servings of grain products, including cereal, pasta, rice, bread, muffins, rolls and crackers, should be offered every day. Offer $1/4$ cup of the cooked grains, $1/2$ bread serving or a couple of crackers.
- Two servings of fruit or fruit juice each day are necessary. Each serving should be about 3 ounces. (Fruit is better than fruit juice.)
- Provide her with three servings of vegetables every day. Each serving should be about 3 ounces.
- Two servings of fish, turkey, chicken, beef, pork, eggs or lentils are adequate. Offer her 1 ounce of meat, 1 egg or $1/4$ cup of lentils.

Some Useful Feeding Tips for this Age

- At this age, it's common for baby to eat heartily at one meal, then not want to eat much at all at the next.
- Vary the tastes and textures of the foods you feed your baby. It makes meals more fun and interesting for her.
- Your growing baby *needs* regular meals and snacks. She is extremely busy and uses a lot of energy. Snacks provide her the energy she needs to keep going. Give

her at least three small snacks a day, in addition to her regular meals.

- When you travel with baby, take foods and snacks that don't need to be kept cold. Crackers, dry-cereal pieces, juices, bread and fruits are good choices.
- When you eat in a restaurant, share a few bites of your food with baby. It's a good change for her, and she may be more interested in eating something new and different.

Baby May Be Feeding Herself

- By the time baby is nearly 1 year old, she should be able to feed herself fairly well.
- She may be able to carry a spoonful of food to her mouth without too much trouble. However, she may spill a lot because her wrist action is not yet fully developed.
- If you try to help her eat, she may resist you, even if it's something she likes. She really does want to do it herself!
- She may be holding a cup quite steadily. And she can drink from it all by herself.
- Allow her to practice eating and drinking without much interference from you. She needs to master these important tasks.
- Stand by with cleaning cloths, and be ready to clean up the mess afterward.

Calorie Check

Do you know how many calories your baby should be eating now to get all the nutrients she needs? According to the AAP, there's a formula you can use to figure out how many calories she needs each day: Multiply her height in inches by the number 40. If she's 31 inches tall, she should consume about 1,240 calories every day.

Snacks Can Be Very Important

- By around 1 year old, your baby may be eating less than she has in the past.
- She may need snacks to help balance her nutrient intake.
- They can provide her with the energy she needs to play and to grow.
- In addition to her regular meals, give her three snacks a day.
- Make them nutritious and delicious! Choose from the following:
    - ~ yogurt—plain is best
    - ~ cheese, thinly sliced
    - ~ baby teething crackers
    - ~ saltine crackers
    - ~ graham crackers
    - ~ small pieces of easily chewed fruit, such as bananas
    - ~ a half slice of bread
    - ~ fruit juice, diluted one-to-one with water

~ pretzels
~ frozen juice pops
~ pudding
~ a small piece of bagel
~ a milkshake
~ oat-circle cereal pieces
~ cut-up raisins

Keep Feeding Baby Food?

You may wonder if you should stop offering baby food at any particular age and switch to "people food."

- As long as you've introduced your baby to finger foods by this time (and she's doing all right with them), it's OK for her to still eat some baby food.
- At this age, you might want to offer her a grown-up version of her baby food. For example, if she loves baby applesauce, switch to a regular one that is fairly smooth.
- When you offer her food that is for everyone, choose foods without sugar or other additives, when possible. She doesn't need anything extra in her food.

Does It Have to Be Cow's Milk?

- When baby turns 1, she will probably be ready to begin drinking milk.
- You may be wondering if cow's milk is the only type of milk you can offer her.

- There are other kinds of milk you may give her. However, check with your pediatrician before you offer her *anything* beyond formula.
- He or she may have specific advice in regard to your baby.
- In addition to cow's milk, your choices include the following.
  - ~ *Goat's milk.* It has a tangy taste. It is deficient in vitamin B_{12} and folacin. It may cause an allergic reaction in a child who is sensitive to cow's milk.
  - ~ *Soy milk.* It can be used as an alternative to cow's milk. It should be fortified with vitamin D and calcium.
  - ~ *Rice milk.* It can also be used as an alternative to cow's milk. It should be fortified with vitamin D and calcium.

Why Have We Waited to Give Her Cow's Milk?

You have been advised not to give your baby cow's milk until the end of her first year for various reasons.

- Her digestive system hasn't been mature enough to handle it.
- Her kidneys and digestive system could not safely process the proteins and minerals in whole milk.
- If you give her cow's milk before she turns 1 year old, you might cause mild damage to the lining of her intestines. This could result in problems.
- Your baby should drink *whole cow's milk* for the next year, until she's 2.

FROM A MOM'S PERSPECTIVE

My baby was a preemie and had to stay in the hospital for a while. I couldn't feed her anything because she had tubes in her nose. My doctor suggested I pump my breasts and store the milk for when she came home. I followed his suggestion, and my milk came in great. I stored enough so that as soon as she could begin sucking from a bottle, she had my breast milk to drink. And she did real well breastfeeding when she came home, too. Breastfeeding her helped us bond because we hadn't been able to get very close to her while she was in the hospital. *Debby*

- She needs the fat and calories to grow and to develop.
- After she turns 2, until she is 5, you can gradually make the transition from whole cow's milk to low-fat or skim milk. Don't make the change too abruptly.

Baby's Interest in Food

- Your baby's interest in eating as she nears 1 year old may be almost nonexistent.
- Don't become anxious about the situation. Don't expect her to eat three well-balanced meals every day.
- Spend your energies on other activities, such as playing with her and helping her learn about her world.
- If she skips a food group one day, offer her more of that food group the next day.
- Provide her with nutritious meals and snacks each day.

Safety at Mealtimes

You want to protect your baby while she's eating. To protect her from getting hurt, consider the following suggestions.

- She's not ready for a fork yet, so don't give her one to feed herself or to play with.
- Don't let her walk or run when she's eating something.
- Don't let her walk or run while she's carrying any utensils.
- Use plastic for safety—plastic spoons, plastic dishes, plastic cups.

- Over the long run, she'll get the nutrition she needs.
- And before long, she'll probably begin eating again.
- If you are concerned, discuss it with your baby's doctor at her next well-baby checkup.

Raisins and Tooth Decay

Your baby is just starting to get a mouthful of teeth, and you want to protect them. One way to do that is to brush her teeth every time she eats raisins.

- Raisins are chewed longer than most other snacks. They also stick to the teeth. This exposes tooth enamel to mouth acids for long periods, which can lead to tooth decay.
- Brushing her teeth after she eats raisins removes the problem.
- If you can't brush her teeth, rinse her mouth out with water to help wash raisin bits out of her teeth.

Nutrients Your Baby Needs

- Research has shown that during your child's first 2 years, she needs to get about 40% of her daily calories from fat sources.

- Studies have shown that at 6 months of age, a little over 40% of calories come from fat. However, by age 1 year, this percentage has dropped to about 30%.

- A deficit in the amount of fat she eats can be unhealthy.

- Often a baby eats what her parents eat. If you are eating low-fat foods, you may believe the same foods are OK to feed baby. They're not!

- If you drink low-fat or skim milk, you may want to give the same product to your baby. This results in less-than-desirable percentages of fat in the diet.

- Don't limit your child's fat intake until after she turns 2. At that point, you can begin to decrease it gradually.

- Until she's quite a bit older, don't feed her fat-reduced foods.

- Many babies don't get enough vitamin D or zinc either. Some low-fat and fat-free products aren't vitamin-D fortified, such as cheese and yogurt.

- Often parents don't realize this, so they feed baby these foods without offering others that do contain vitamin D. Good sources of vitamin D include eggs, fortified milk and butter.

- Zinc is found in beef, pork and poultry. Children may resist eating these foods. Encourage your child to eat them. Two or three tablespoons a day of beef, pork, poultry or eggs provide her with enough zinc.

The End of Baby's 1st Year

You've had quite a year, moving from breast milk or formula to baby's eating table food with the rest of the family. It's probably been an exciting year for the many other things that have happened to you as a family. As baby becomes a toddler, keep nutrition at the top of the list of good things to do for her. Her entire future rests on the good start she gets now.

Part V: Situations and Problems that May Arise

In this section, we have listed, in alphabetical order, some situations and problems related to feeding that you may experience with your baby during the first year. Look up the following if you have any questions or concerns:

- acid reflux
- amebic dysentery
- botulism
- celiac disease
- choking on formula or breast milk
- constipation
- dehydration
- diarrhea
- preventing E. coli
- failure to thrive
- fecal impaction
- food allergies
- food poisoning
- gassiness
- gastroenteritis
- giardiasis
- lactose intolerance
- malabsorption syndrome

- obesity
- tapeworm
- thrush
- vomiting

Acid Reflux

Acid reflux, also called *gastroesophageal reflux disease (GERD)*, occurs when the contents of baby's tummy bubble up into the esophagus. This can irritate baby's throat and cause him to pull away from the bottle or breast while he's feeding. He may refuse to feed for a bit but then want to feed again immediately.

- Acid reflux can occur at any age, and nearly everyone experiences it at some time.
- It is the frequency and persistence of the problem that make it abnormal.
- In a baby, it is usually a mild problem that improves by about 1 year of age.
- Symptoms of acid reflux include the following:
  - ~ spitting up
  - ~ vomiting (can be forceful)
  - ~ weight loss
  - ~ gagging or choking at the end of a feeding
  - ~ respiratory problems
  - ~ irritability
  - ~ hiccups

~ coughing

~ apnea (stops breathing for a bit)

- If it's a mild case, burping baby and holding him upright for about 30 minutes after he eats helps resolve the problem.
- Give him small, frequent feedings.
- Burp him more frequently than you have been.
- Change the position of his infant seat or the head of his crib so it is more upright.
- Sometimes adding rice cereal to formula can help. Do *not* do this unless your pediatrician says it's OK.
- If the problem is more severe, discuss it with your pediatrician. He or she may want to treat baby with medication.
- Call baby's doctor if he vomits excessively, loses weight or has respiratory problems.
- If you see blood in the vomit or baby has apnea spells (he stops breathing for a short time), contact your pediatrician.
- Medications may be prescribed to decrease the amount of acid in the stomach contents or to promote gastric emptying.
- If the problem is serious, nasogastric feedings (putting a tube through the nose into the stomach) may be necessary for a baby who has severe reflux.
- Acid reflux could result in his failure to thrive.
- Surgery may be required if a baby has severe complications, such as recurring aspiration pneumonia,

apnea and severe irritation or inflammation of the esophagus, or if medication doesn't work.

Amebic Dysentery

Amebic dysentery, also called *amebiasis* or *entamebiasis*, is a parasitic infection of the large bowel or colon.

- It is spread when food is contaminated with human feces.
- It occurs most often when food handlers don't wash their hands after using the bathroom.
- Flies and insects can also contaminate foods. Some raw fruits and vegetables fertilized with human feces or washed in polluted water may be contaminated.
- The problem can occur at any age.
- Symptoms of the problem include:
  - ~ diarrhea
  - ~ bloating of the abdomen
  - ~ nausea
  - ~ vomiting
  - ~ fever
  - ~ foul-smelling stools
  - ~ gas
  - ~ cramping and pain in the abdomen
  - ~ blood or mucus in the stool
  - ~ irritability
- Avoid the problem by washing hands thoroughly after using the bathroom or changing baby's dirty diaper.

- Wash raw fruits and vegetables well before preparing or serving.
- Cover food to keep flies and other insects from contaminating it.
- Kitchen counters should be cleaned with soap and water, bleach or some other disinfecting agent.
- Take care in preparing and storing food.
- Call the doctor if your baby has symptoms of amebic dysentery.
- The problem becomes more serious if baby experiences an increase in diarrhea, has blood in his stools or pain increases.
- Occasionally, antibiotics are prescribed.
- Rest and fluid replacement are also good measures.
- If your baby gets amebic dysentery, use extra care in the future with food preparation and storage.
- Practice good hand washing. When you can't wash your hands with soap and water, consider using antibacterial gel hand cleaners that do not require any water.

Botulism

Botulism is a severe form of food poisoning. The toxins that cause botulism are found in the soil and improperly canned meats and vegetables.

- In infants, exposure to botulism most often comes from raw honey and other uncooked foods.

FROM A MOM'S PERSPECTIVE

I could tell that Bill wanted me to breastfeed our baby. We talked about it before we even got pregnant. He said his mother had nursed him and his three brothers as long as she could. At first I was surprised that he even had an opinion, but his support made a big difference to me. Even though I was the one doing it, his interest made me feel like we were doing it together. *Liz*

- Symptoms of botulism include:
  - ~ vomiting
  - ~ diarrhea
  - ~ nausea
  - ~ abdominal pain
  - ~ dizziness
  - ~ problems sucking, swallowing or eating
  - ~ dry mouth
  - ~ weakness
  - ~ lethargy
  - ~ weak cry
  - ~ constipation (in infants)
- If you believe your baby has botulism, identify others who are sick. Determine whether they ate the same foods or were exposed in some other way.
- Call the doctor immediately or go to the emergency room if you believe your baby has botulism.
- You will be directed by your baby's doctor or an emergency-medicine physician as to treatment. It

can include botulism antitoxin, which is given by injection.
· Bed rest and fluids may be prescribed. Baby may also be admitted to the hospital for I.V. therapy.

Celiac Disease

Celiac disease is an allergic condition that is triggered by gluten, a protein found in many grains and cereals.
· About 1 in 250 people suffer from the problem.
· The disease affects the small intestine, so it cannot absorb some nutrients.
· The problem can occur any time from infancy through early childhood.
· It usually occurs when baby begins eating cereal and bread.
· Symptoms of celiac disease include:
  ~ weight loss or slow weight gain after adding cereal to his diet
  ~ poor appetite
  ~ diarrhea
  ~ foul-smelling stools
  ~ frequent gas
  ~ swollen abdomen
  ~ abdominal pain
  ~ mouth ulcers
  ~ baby's skin is pale in color
  ~ tendency to bleed easily

- If you suspect your baby may have celiac disease, carefully monitor his diet.
- Document any changes you see as you introduce or withhold foods.
- One study showed the risk of celiac disease was reduced by nearly 40% if a baby continued breastfeeding while beginning solid foods that contained gluten, such as bread and cereal.
- If your baby has many of the above symptoms, and there is a family history of the problem (most forms are inherited), call your pediatrician.
- If symptoms don't decrease within 3 weeks of changing baby's diet, your pediatrician will probably want to see him.
- It's also serious if your baby doesn't regain lost weight, or he fails to grow and to develop as expected.
- Call if a fever develops.
- Your doctor may prescribe oral cortisone drugs to reduce baby's inflammatory response during a severe attack.

Choking on Formula or Breast Milk

Occasionally a baby chokes on formula, breast milk or mucus.
- It's a common occurrence and one you can handle easily.
- When it happens, turn baby's head to the side and put his head a little lower than his body.

- If you need to, use a cloth, your clean finger or a bulb syringe to help clear any fluid from his mouth.

Constipation

When a baby is constipated, he has difficulty passing bowel movements, infrequent bowel movements or sluggish bowel action.

- The condition occurs more often in older infants, when baby begins eating solids or with other dietary changes.
- The main symptom of the problem is baby's difficulty passing dry, hard stools.
- This may be accompanied by abdominal pain, which decreases after a large bowel movement.
- Baby may go several days between bowel movements.
- You may notice stool is blood streaked.
- If your baby is breastfeeding and goes a few days between bowel movements, this is *not* considered constipation.
- If your younger baby seems constipated, use a rectal thermometer lubricated with petroleum jelly to stimulate the passage of stools. Gently place the thermometer in the rectum, then remove it.
- If your baby is older and eating solids, offer him lots of fluid and diluted juice. Apple juice often has a laxative effect.
- Increase the fiber content of baby's diet.

- Most cases resolve with time if they are caused by a change in diet.
- Call your pediatrician if the above measures don't work.
- Call the office if baby's constipation is accompanied by severe abdominal pain or vomiting.
- Do *not* use any medication to relieve constipation without first consulting the doctor.
- Your doctor may suggest an enema or a mild laxative for baby.
- If constipation becomes chronic or serious, testing may be ordered to determine the cause.

Dehydration

Dehydration results when baby doesn't take in enough fluids or loses too much fluid from his body.

- It can occur if your baby is not breastfeeding properly or if you are not producing enough milk.
- It may also arise in cases of vomiting and diarrhea.
- Dehydration occasionally occurs when a baby becomes overheated and does not receive enough fluid to compensate for his overheating. When this occurs, it usually happens in hot summer months.
- Dehydration should be a concern if baby's coloring becomes grayish, his mucous membranes are dry, urination has deceased, there is an absence of tears, his fontanel (the soft spot on the top of his head) is

sunken in and he has a rapid pulse and respiration. Your baby may also be very lethargic.

- You should be changing a wet diaper six to eight times a day, and your baby should have three or more stools each day.
- If you notice these symptoms, and you are breastfeeding, carefully monitor your baby's feeding patterns.
- Make sure you can see or hear him gulping milk when he feeds.
- Does he seem satisfied after a nursing session? A full baby will be content.
- To avoid dehydration, keep baby out of the sun so he doesn't get sunburned or overheated.
- In hot weather, make sure he has plenty of fluids. Give him water *only* when advised to do so by your pediatrician.
- Dress baby appropriately.
- Call your pediatrician immediately if your baby has any of the following symptoms:
  ~ hasn't had a wet diaper in 6 to 8 eight hours
  ~ has been vomiting for more than 12 hours
  ~ has passed more than eight diarrheal stools in 8 hours
  ~ has a dry mouth and cries without tears (newborns may not show tears with crying)
  ~ your baby is inconsolable
  ~ your baby seems unusually drowsy or sleepy, or doesn't respond to you
  ~ your baby has a sunken fontanel

- Your baby's doctor may recommend oral rehydration in mild to moderate cases. In this situation, baby is given a prepared solution with electrolytes. Frequent, small amounts are fed to him over a period of time.
- If the situation is severe, a pediatrician may admit the baby to the hospital.
- I.V. fluids are given to replace lost fluids.
- Accurate measurements of fluid intake and output are also recorded.

Diarrhea

When your baby gets diarrhea, it's not an illness. It's a *symptom* of a medical problem, usually one involving the gastrointestinal area.

- Diarrhea is more common in older infants, although babies of almost any age can have diarrhea.
- If your baby has more than five loose, liquid or watery bowel movements in one day, and he is otherwise healthy, he has diarrhea.
- Loose stools may be accompanied by irritation or diaper rash around the anus.
- He may also be fussy and/or have cramplike pains in his lower abdomen.
- In some cases, he may run a fever.
- When your baby has diarrhea, the most important thing you can do is increase his fluid intake.

- Don't give him *any medications,* unless your pediatrician tells you to do so.
- If baby is eating solids, decrease the amount you feed him.
- Contact your pediatrician if you notice any of the following.
  - ~ Diarrhea lasts longer than 36 hours.
  - ~ There is blood in the stool.
  - ~ Baby's temperature is higher than 102F.
  - ~ He isn't feeding well or refuses to eat.
  - ~ He appears dehydrated—his mouth is dry or urination decreases.
  - ~ You see worms or other parasites in his stool.
- Your doctor probably won't prescribe medication to treat the diarrhea if baby is less than a year old.
- He or she may recommend you stop feeding him his regular diet of formula or breast milk and solids. In some cases, you will be advised on how often to feed baby and the amounts to give him.
- You may be advised to give him an electrolyte solution to replace the electrolytes he has lost.

Preventing E. coli

E. coli is a bacteria that is present in the alimentary canal (the digestive tube from the mouth to the anus) of humans and other animals.

FROM A MOM'S PERSPECTIVE

I am so proud of myself for nursing Eric. It wasn't easy. I had to go back to work 6 weeks after he was born. Pumping and saving milk was a challenge and rarely convenient, but I did it. I found people at work were very supportive; they even gave me my own spot in the refrigerator where I could store the milk I pumped. *Alice*

- This bacteria is responsible for infections, such as urinary-tract infections, stomach aches and diarrhea.
- A baby can be exposed to E. coli in many ways, including the environment and foods you feed him.
- If you take your baby into a swimming pool that is used by a lot of people, you risk exposure. Some kids urinate in the pool. Others swim with dirty diapers. When they do, microorganisms can wash into the water. Chlorine may not kill all these organisms, so if baby drinks the water, he can be exposed. Protect your baby when you go swimming.
- Take the following steps to protect baby from E. coli when you are preparing and serving foods.
  ~ Wash your hands, utensils and any other items that come in contact with raw meat or raw poultry.
  ~ If you prepare beef, cook it until it is well done or at least 160F internally.
  ~ Beverages should be pasteurized, if necessary.
  ~ If you prepare chicken, cook it until the internal temperature reaches 180F.

~ Never place cooked meat on a plate that was used for raw meat unless it has been thoroughly washed with soap and water.
~ Wash all fruits and vegetables before serving raw. Manure on the outside peel could cause contamination.

Failure to Thrive

If your baby does not gain enough weight, his doctor may be concerned about failure to thrive.

- The problem may also be suspected if baby was gaining weight then suddenly stops for no apparent reason.
- Increase the frequency of the feedings you give baby.
- Feed him for longer periods, too.
- Try to get him to take more at each feeding—don't rush him to eat. Setting up a schedule of feedings may help increase his caloric intake.
- Consultation with a dietician or breastfeeding (lactation) specialist may offer you additional strategies to try.
- If your baby is not getting enough breast milk from nursing, you may be advised to supplement with formula or pumped breast milk.
- Contact your pediatrician if this situation occurs. He or she will want to know about it because weight gain is extremely important to baby during the 1st year.

- In addition to extra or supplemental feedings, baby's doctor may advise you to give baby vitamin or nutritional supplements.
- When the above measures don't solve the problem, baby may need to be admitted to the hospital for further evaluation.
- I.V. therapy may be needed.

Fecal Impaction

When a baby suffers from fecal impaction, he has a large amount of stool he cannot pass. His intestines are overloaded.

- It's a form of constipation and can be very uncomfortable.
- It can occur at any age.
- Symptoms of fecal impaction include the following:
  ~ no bowel movements
  ~ hard mass in the lower left abdomen
  ~ abdominal discomfort
  ~ irritability
  ~ poor feeding
- If you believe your baby is suffering from fecal impaction, increase the amount of fluid you offer him to avoid dehydration.
- Contact your pediatrician. He or she may want you to bring baby into the office.
- You may be advised to give the baby an enema to deal with the constipation.

Food Allergies

A food allergy is hypersensitivity to a particular food. The most common causes of food allergies include cow's milk, wheat, eggs, peanuts, seafood, some fruits, tomatoes and some legumes.

- Food allergy can occur at any age but usually does not occur until a child begins eating solid foods or when he begins drinking cow's milk.
- Occasionally a baby is allergic to formula made of cow's milk and must be put on a different type of formula.
- Although a food allergy can occur at any time, the chance of your baby having one is relatively low—only about 6%.
- It's important to know the signs and symptoms of a food allergy. As you add new foods to your baby's diet, make note of new foods you offer him.
- If he has any reactions, you'll have a better idea of what may be causing it.
- Different allergies may cause different kinds of symptoms.
- Symptoms of a food allergy include the following:
  - ~ bloating and gassiness
  - ~ nausea
  - ~ vomiting
  - ~ itching
  - ~ skin rash
  - ~ crying

- ~ fatigue
- ~ feeding problems
- ~ congested nose or a runny nose, with a thin, clear discharge
- ~ sandpaperlike red rash on the face
- ~ watery, itchy eyes
- ~ upset stomach
- ~ diarrhea or mucus in the stools
- ~ red rash around the anus
- ~ fussiness
- Call your pediatrician if you believe baby has a food allergy.

You Can Help Avoid Food Allergies

- To help eliminate problems, follow your pediatrician's instructions for adding new foods to your baby's diet.
- Keep track of *every* new food you give baby.
- Introduce new foods one at a time. Wait to see if baby has any reactions before you offer him another new food.
- Rice products cause fewer allergy problems than wheat products.
- Don't give him any peanut products before age 3.
- If your baby displays any symptoms of a food allergy, eliminate foods you can identify that might be causing the problem.
- Foods that most often cause allergies include egg whites, cow's milk and some citrus fruits and juices.

Wait until baby is at least 9 months old before you offer him any citrus juice.

- Discuss the situation with your baby's doctor if you or your partner have a food allergy. It might affect the types of food you feed him.

- In addition, research has found that if a mother breastfeeds her baby, *her* diet is important. If she eats a diet higher in carbohydrates and lower in total and saturated fats, baby has a lower chance of developing allergies by age 1.

- If baby has a skin rash, bathe him with a mild, nondrying soap. Use a lubricating cream to decrease redness or itching. Avoid frequent bathing.

- Call the doctor if any reaction is severe. Call immediately if your baby develops any breathing difficulties!

- Contact your pediatrician if a rash looks infected or if the treatment you have tried is not working.

Treating Food Allergies

- If you believe your baby has a food allergy, try to identify the problem food.

- Don't give the food to him again without first discussing it with your pediatrician.

- Increase the amount of fluid you give him. Decrease solid food until he feels better.

- Treatment for a food allergy is avoidance of the food.

- However, it may be difficult to identify the food causing the problems. In this case, allergy testing can be done.

- If you are breastfeeding, nurse your baby for at least 6 months if there is a history of food allergies in the family. Feeding for this length of time helps some babies avoid the problem.
- Many children eventually outgrow food allergies.
- *Be aware:* If your baby is allergic to eggs, be sure your pediatrician and any other doctor who treats him is aware of it. Certain vaccines are egg-based. You will need to take precautions with these vaccines.

Food Poisoning

The term *food poisoning* is used to describe an illness resulting from eating a food that contains poisonous substances.

- True food poisoning includes poisoning from mushrooms, shellfish, insecticides and milk from cows that have eaten poisonous plants.
- The food-rotting process can also poison foods.
- It would be extremely rare in a baby that is not yet eating solid foods to be exposed to contaminated foods.
- Food poisoning usually occurs in those who eat solids.
- Symptoms of food poisoning include the following:
  ~ nausea
  ~ vomiting
  ~ severe abdominal cramps
  ~ profuse diarrhea
- If your baby exhibits any of the above symptoms, offer him lots of fluid to help prevent dehydration.

- Let him rest.
- Call the doctor if your baby develops a fever or signs of dehydration.
- Medical treatment is usually unnecessary.
- Symptoms usually improve within 24 hours.

Gassiness

Problems with gassiness or flatulence can occur at any age.
- It is more common once baby starts eating solid foods, between 4 and 6 months of age.
- Symptoms of excessive gas include:
  ~ abdominal pain
  ~ bloated or distended abdomen
  ~ fussiness
  ~ frequent passing of gas
- If you are breastfeeding, make note of foods you have eaten. Some of them could cause baby to be gassy. Avoid these foods in the future.
- If baby is eating solids, keep track of the foods he eats that might cause him to be uncomfortable.
- Most of the time you won't have to call your doctor about this problem. It usually resolves on its own.
- In a few cases, gas may be caused by a digestive problem.
- If baby has diarrhea, vomits, cries inconsolably and suffers from bloating, call your doctor. Baby may have lactose intolerance, may be allergic to his formula or may suffer from some other problem.

- Also call the doctor if you notice any of the following symptoms:
  - ~ severe abdominal pain that is not relieved by passing gas
  - ~ baby is still uncomfortable after using the above treatments
  - ~ he has a fever
  - ~ you notice any blood in his stools
- If baby's problem is severe, your pediatrician may prescribe medications to help eliminate gas in the intestines.
- Do *not* give him any medication before consulting the doctor.
- If the problem becomes chronic or very severe, further testing may be done to find its cause.

Ways to Relieve Baby's Gas

- A baby often swallows air when he eats, so it's not unusual for him to have some gas.
- Burping often takes care of the problem, but when it doesn't, you may need to try some other things.
- Use a different burping position. Lay him face down on your lap, and pat his back. Or sit him on your lap while you rub his back.
- Stop in the middle of his feeding and burp him. Burp him again when he finishes.
- Don't let him cry for long periods. When he cries, he gulps in air, which can cause gas.

- When you feed him, keep him upright, at least at a 30° angle. This helps food go down more easily, and he'll swallow less air.

- If you use a bottle, be sure the nipple is the right size. Too much milk going through too fast or sucking too hard on a nipple with an opening that is too small can cause him to swallow air.

- Go modern—use an angled bottle, use disposable plastic liners that collapse as baby sucks or buy a nipple that lets you change the flow. In all cases, baby will take in less air.

- Lay him on his tummy on top of a hot-water bottle or a warm (not hot!) heating pad for a short time. Massage his tummy.

Gastroenteritis

Gastroenteritis is an inflammation of the stomach and intestinal tract, resulting in irritation or infection of the digestive tract.

- It can be contagious and can occur at any age.
- Symptoms of gastroenteritis include the following:
  ~ vomiting
  ~ diarrhea
  ~ irritability
  ~ poor appetite
  ~ fever
- You can try various treatments at home.

- Fluids are necessary, but the bowel also needs to rest.
- Offer a clear liquid diet for the first day or two.
- In young infants, a commercial electrolyte solution, such as Pedialyte, can be used.
- In older infants, clear liquid is "anything you can see through."
- For a child under 1 year, give 1/2 ounce of fluid every 20 to 30 minutes. Consult your pediatrician before using this treatment.
- When a child has been free of diarrhea for 1 day, a bland diet may be offered. This includes bananas, rice, applesauce, tea and toast. This is called the *BRATT diet.* (You probably want to avoid giving tea at this age.)
- If diarrhea doesn't recur within 2 hours after eating the BRATT diet, continue feeding bland foods for 24 hours. Gradually work back to a normal diet.
- *Caution:* Do *not* use any nonprescription antidiarrheal drugs without first consulting your baby's doctor.
- If your baby has symptoms of gastroenteritis, you may be able to take care of the problem at home. However, you should call the doctor if:
  ~ rectal temperature rises to 103F or higher
  ~ your child shows signs of dehydration
  ~ symptoms don't improve in 48 hours, despite treatment
  ~ your baby is under 2 months old
- Hospitalization may be recommended for I.V. hydration, if baby is dehydrated.
- The condition should improve in 48 hours.

My older kids were my biggest support and help when I nursed my youngest daughter. I could tell it was important to them that I breastfeed. They helped me with things around the house so I could have the time to spend with the baby. Nursing was a "family thing" they took pride in. *Lilly*

Giardiasis

Giardiasis is an infection that causes inflammation of the bowel. It is caused by a parasite found in contaminated food or contaminated water.

- It can occur at any age but is most common in older infants and children.
- Symptoms of giardiasis include the following:
  - ~ diarrhea
  - ~ fever
  - ~ nausea
  - ~ weakness
  - ~ gas
  - ~ belching
  - ~ vomiting
  - ~ abdominal cramps
  - ~ greasy, bad-smelling stools
- Prevention of this problem is your best bet.
- Don't let your baby have water that could be contaminated. Use water from normal water supplies. If you

don't know whether water is safe, boil it for 5 minutes.

- Because of nausea, vomiting and diarrhea, give your baby lots of fluids to avoid dehydration.
- Don't use over-the-counter medications for diarrhea or nausea and vomiting, unless advised by your pediatrician.
- Call the doctor if your baby has symptoms of giardiasis.
- It's important to let your pediatrician know if baby has a fever, severe abdominal pain or is dehydrated.
- Your doctor may do laboratory studies of stools to detect parasites.
- Usually tests are done three times before being considered negative.
- An antiparasitic drug, such as metronidazole, furazolidone or quinacrine, may be prescribed. These drugs are very effective.
- In severe cases, when baby suffers from dehydration or malabsorption, hospitalization may be necessary for I.V. hydration and nutrition supplementation.

Lactose Intolerance

When a person suffers from lactose intolerance, also called *lactase deficiency* or *milk intolerance,* he has a problem digesting cow's milk or other milk products.

- The condition is caused by a deficiency in, or the lack of, the enzyme lactase. Lactase is necessary to digest all milk products other than breast milk.
- Lactose intolerance can occur at any age. Some infants are born with this disorder.
- Symptoms of lactose intolerance include:
  ~ diarrhea
  ~ failure to thrive
  ~ failure to gain weight
  ~ diaper rash
  ~ gas
  ~ stomach pain
  ~ nausea
  ~ vomiting
- Lactose intolerance is more common in some races of people than others. Asians, Blacks and Native Americans have a higher incidence of lactose intolerance. It also runs in families.
- While you're pregnant, seriously consider breastfeeding your baby if you or the baby's father have a family history of lactose intolerance.
- Be alert for problems with formula, especially if it is cow-milk based.
- When baby turns 1 year old, look for signs of lactose intolerance when you switch him to regular cow's milk.
- If lactose intolerance does not run in your family, you may have to become a detective. When baby has prob-

lems such as those listed above, try to identify what might be causing them.

- Call your pediatrician if you believe your baby has lactose intolerance, especially after switching to cow's milk from formula or breast milk.
- If baby suffers from persistent diarrhea or vomiting, or if he doesn't gain weight, let his doctor know.
- The best treatment is to change baby's diet.
- Do not give him any cow's milk or products that contain, or are made from, cow's milk.
- A supplement (lactase) can be added to milk and milk-containing foods to help deal with the problem.
- If the condition is present at birth, and you choose not to nurse, you may be advised to give baby a soybean-based formula.

Malabsorption Syndrome

Some babies suffer from malabsorption syndrome. They do not absorb enough nutrients from the food they eat.

- When a baby has malabsorption, he loses weight, displays physical weakness and has gas and diarrhea, often with foul-smelling bowel movements.
- The problem can arise from, or be associated with, infections, lactase deficiency or antibiotic treatment.
- If you believe your baby may be experiencing this problem, observe his bowel movements. Make note of

their amount and regularity. Indicate whether stools are particularly foul smelling.

- Increase the number of times you feed him each day, and offer him more at each feeding.
- Call your doctor for advice. He or she may want to see the baby, especially if there is no obvious reason for the problem, such as baby has been taking antibiotics.
- Your physician may change baby's diet and/or prescribe vitamins.
- Further testing may also be recommended.

Obesity

Although a child of any age can be extremely overweight, the term is rarely used to describe a newborn, infant or young baby.

- Most babies do not become extremely overweight in their first year, unless there is a medical reason for it.
- Obesity is defined as being at least 20% above a person's desirable weight for his or her height.
- With babies and young children, there is a range of average weights *and* heights for infants and young children. The key is the height-to-weight comparison.
- At each office visit with your pediatrician, he or she will weigh your baby.
- Your doctor will be able to tell you how your baby's height and weight compare to other children of the same age.

- Babies develop, grow and gain weight at different rates. Your baby's doctor will help you understand what's normal for your baby.
- Do *not* restrict your baby's food and formula or breast milk, even if you think he's too big.
- He needs the vitamins, minerals and other nutrients from the food he eats to develop physically *and* mentally!
- Follow the instructions your pediatrician has given you with regard to feeding and vitamin supplements.
- If you are concerned, discuss the situation with your baby's doctor at one of baby's regularly scheduled well-baby visits.
- Your pediatrician can provide you with specific instructions regarding your child's food intake.

Tapeworm

A tapeworm is a parasite that can live in a person's intestines.

- A person can get a tapeworm from eating raw or undercooked meat that contains the tapeworm larvae.
- It is not contagious from one person to another. To avoid the problem, do *not* eat or feed other family members raw or undercooked meat.
- Symptoms of a tapeworm include the following:
  ~ diarrhea
  ~ tenderness of the upper abdomen
  ~ failure to thrive

~ weight loss
~ listlessness
~ poor feeding
~ irritability
~ worms or eggs in the stool
- Call the doctor if you notice an increase in diarrhea or blood in the stools.
- Antiparasitic medication may be prescribed.

Thrush

Thrush is a yeast infection of the mouth, also called *Candida albicans.*

- The problem is a common infection and isn't serious, although the initial appearance may be startling.
- It often looks like curdled milk in baby's mouth or on his lips.
- Thrush occurs most often in newborns and infants.
- Thrush has been seen as early as a few hours following birth.
- It may be passed from mother to baby as baby passes through the birth canal, if the delivering mother has a yeast infection.
- It may also be passed from baby to mother's nipples during breastfeeding. See the discussion on page 168.
- The most common symptom is white patches or "plaques" in the baby's mouth. Patches may be found on gums, tongue, cheeks, lips or the soft palate. They

are white or cream colored and may be raised; they are not usually painful. Baby's mouth may also be dry.

- If you are nursing, you may contract thrush from your baby.
- Your nipples may suddenly be sore, red, itchy and burn. Deep shooting pain around your nipples after feeding is another warning sign.
- If you believe you have a yeast infection on your breasts, take care of it.
- If you are bottlefeeding, sterilize nipples and bottles by boiling them. If these items are not sterilized, baby can become reinfected.
- Sterilize pacifiers by boiling them for a few minutes. Wash any toys baby chews on—use soap and water or put them in the washing machine or dishwasher, if it is safe to do so.
- Antibiotics can also trigger the infection. However, if your baby is taking antibiotics and gets thrush, don't stop giving him any medication without consulting your doctor.
- Call the baby's doctor if he is feeding poorly, if he is dehydrated or if he loses weight.
- If he develops a fever or has signs of a secondary bacterial infection, with redness or bleeding, contact your pediatrician.
- Your doctor may prescribe an oral antifungal medication for baby and an antifungal cream for you.
- Keep up baby's fluid intake.

FROM A MOM'S PERSPECTIVE

I had trouble breastfeeding my first baby when I came home from the hospital. I had no idea what to do, and he was so hungry all the time! He just cried and cried. I was at my wit's end when a good friend told me about the La Leche League. I called them, and they sent a very nice lady out to my house to help me. She spent a lot of time showing me things and talking with me, and she kept in touch with me after she left. She said she wanted to check to make sure I was doing all right. I bless her for all the help she gave me. Without the La Leche League, I don't know what I would have done! *Pat*

Vomiting

Vomiting is usually a symptom, not an illness. It's a *sign* that something might be making baby feel ill.

- Vomiting usually results from stomach or intestinal upset.
- It can also be a symptom of other problems, including appendicitis, pneumonia, strep throat or meningitis.
- Vomiting may occur after ingestion of a medication or chemical.
- Vomiting is different from when baby "spits up." That usually occurs after a feeding, and he spits up only a little bit of the total amount he has taken in.
- When your baby vomits, he expels the contents of his stomach.

- Other symptoms that may accompany vomiting include fever, listlessness, poor feeding, coughing, constipation, diarrhea or dehydration.
- When baby vomits, try to identify the cause. Is he getting a cold or the flu?
- Don't force him to eat, but offer him liquids to avoid dehydration.
- If your baby vomits repeatedly or if vomiting lasts more than a few hours, call your physician.
- If your baby is under 6 months old, it's especially important to contact your doctor.
- Treatment your doctor may prescribe depends on the cause of the vomiting.
- You may be advised to stop feeding him solids and offer only liquids.
- Medication may also be prescribed, depending on the cause of the vomiting.

Authors' Note to Readers

We are always happy to hear from the readers of our books. You are welcome to address letters to us via our publisher, DaCapo Press, or you may send them to us by email. If you use email, we will probably be able to reply more quickly. Our email address is **yourpregnancy@juno.com**.

When you send us an email, please do not ask us medical questions about your particular situation. We are unable to reply to these letters, except to suggest you discuss your question with your own physician. We are happy to answer general questions about areas we address in our books. We are also happy to clear up any confusion regarding information we present. If you have comments or suggestions for areas to address in future books, we are always glad to receive these suggestions.

If you send us an email, please do not include any attachments. We will not open these because of the problem with viruses. In addition, we ask that you do not add us to any lists for stories, chain letters, prayers, political or other causes, charitable donations or any other lists you can think of.

We will attempt to answer your emails as quickly as possible, but please understand that with all the books we have published, we are kept busy updating them and doing research for new books. In addition, Dr. Curtis sees patients nearly every day. We'll get back to you as soon as we can!

Index

Also by Glade B. Curtis, M.D., M.P.H., OB-GYN, and Judith Schuler, M.S.

***Your Pregnancy
Week by Week, 5th Edition***
ISBN: 1-55561-346-2 (paper)
1-55561-347-0 (cloth)

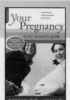

***Your Pregnancy:
Every Woman's Guide***
ISBN: 0-7382-1001-3

***Bouncing Back
After Your Pregnancy***
ISBN: 0-7382-0606-7

***Your Pregnancy
Questions and Answers***
ISBN: 0-7382-1003-X

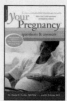

***Your Baby's First Year,
Week by Week***
ISBN: 0-7382-0975-9 (paper)
0-7382-0974-0 (cloth)

***Your Pregnancy
Quick Guide:
Labor and Delivery***
ISBN: 0-7382-0969-4

***Your Pregnancy
for the Father to Be***
ISBN: 0-7382-1002-1

***Your Pregnancy
Quick Guide:
Tests and Procedures***
ISBN: 0-7382-0953-8

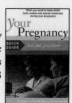

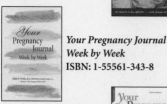

***Your Pregnancy Journal
Week by Week***
ISBN: 1-55561-343-8

***Your Pregnancy Quick Guide:
Nutrition and
Weight Management***
ISBN: 0-7382-0954-6

Your Pregnancy After 35
ISBN: 0-7382-1004-8

***Your Pregnancy
Quick Guide:
Fitness and Exercise***
ISBN: 0-7382-0952-X

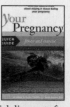

Da Capo Lifelong Books are available wherever books are sold and at special discounts for bulk purchases in the U.S. by corporations, institutions, and other organizations. For more information, please contact the Special Markets Department at the Perseus Books Group, 11 Cambridge Center, Cambridge, MA 02142, or call (800) 255-1514.